PSYCHIATRY

AND

RELIGION

PSYCHIATRY

and

RELIGION

Edited by
JOSHUA LOTH LIEBMAN

Introduction by
ALBERT A. GOLDMAN

Essay Index Reprint Series

 BOOKS FOR LIBRARIES PRESS
FREEPORT, NEW YORK

Copyright, 1948, The Beacon Press

Reprinted 1972 by arrangement with
Mrs. Joshua Loth Liebman

Library of Congress Cataloging in Publication Data

Institute on Religion and Psychiatry, Congregation
    Adath Israel, Boston, 1947.
    Psychiatry and religion.

    (Essay index reprint series)
    1. Pastoral psychology (Judaism) 2. Psycho-
therapy. I. Liebman, Joshua Loth, 1907-1948, ed.
II. Title.
[BM652.5.I6 1947b]   150   72-156666
ISBN 0-8369-2658-7

PRINTED IN THE UNITED STATES OF AMERICA
BY
NEW WORLD BOOK MANUFACTURING CO., INC.
HALLANDALE, FLORIDA 33009

JOSHUA LOTH LIEBMAN
1907–1948

ON JUNE 9, 1948, the entire nation was electrified by the sad news of the untimely passing of Dr. Joshua Loth Liebman. This volume will serve, in a sense, as a monument to his memory, for it reflects his deep interest in the subject of religion and psychiatry and contains within it one of the last chapters he had written in his Book of Life.

While yet a rabbi in Chicago, he began to sense his own inadequacy in dealing with human problems. The courses in practical theology which he had received at the seminary did not enter into the deeper levels of human behavior, and he realized, as all of his colleagues have realized at one time or another, that more profound insights were needed if he were to help the troubled in the solution of their problems.

It was typical of him never to leave a challenge unanswered. His penetrating mind had to follow an idea to its very end. He had to understand all of its ramifications, its nuances, its hidden depths, until he grasped it in crystal-like clarity. As he began to deal with the many personal problems brought him, he recognized that here, too, lay a great challenge, and that he could never be content to be merely a spectator; he had to be a friend and counselor. For years, then, he subjected himself to the rigid discipline of analyzing the depths within himself, exploring the layers of his own personality, digging deep into the recesses of his heart, probing mercilessly into his experiences until he came to fuller recognition of the importance of the teachings of Freud and their meaning for our time. He was one of the first religionists to have made his peace with Freud, and although departing from some interpretations, he regarded the founder of psychoanalysis as one of the great geniuses of the twentieth century and one of the necessary forces for the spiritual redemption of modern man. He recognized that Freudianism did not go far enough, for it left untouched the whole realm of ethical and religious orientation. He realized that man needed ideals and purposes, and that God could not be "analyzed" away in a reasonably friendly universe – a universe by which he was enthralled. If he knew that man had to look within himself, he also understood that man had to be uplifted beyond himself and that man divining his own creative powers could become a co-worker with God for the attainment of a better world.

There were some who regarded his emphasis on Freud as an *idée fixe* but they did not realize that Joshua Loth Liebman could never deal with an idea impassively and detachedly. This does not mean that he did not have an objective, critical evaluation of psychiatry and psychoanalysis; for he did. His keen philosophic mind never allowed him the sinecure of dogmatism. But his passion for the subject was spurred on by his compassion for man. He found in this infant science the promise for a mature society; and he recognized that if man could be given the proper insights into himself, he would know how to turn his "spears into pruning hooks."

His own words should be remembered as an indication of his attitude towards these two fields which he sought to bring into fruitful synthesis: "Wherever religion and psychiatry can work together to take a broken, disunited, disordered personality and bring unity into it, there an act of religion is being performed." Thus spake the scholar and the rabbi.

Dr. Liebman's prominence as one of the pioneers in the harmonization of religion and psychiatry was recently evidenced when he was invited by the American Psychiatric

Association to speak at its Convention in May, 1948. His first publication, *Peace of Mind,* has taken its place among the classic works of the twentieth century and remains an everlasting memorial to his ceaseless quest for truth and to his undiminished reverence for man.

This co-worker with God and brother to man has bequeathed his generation an unforgettable legacy. His disciples, who have been privileged to sit at his feet, will always feel the overwhelming warmth of his intense personality; they will remain fired by his consecrated determination for the achievement of the good life and inspired to acts of goodness by his revered memory.

Zekher tsaddik livrakha

The memory of the righteous is
an eternal blessing.

ALBERT A. GOLDMAN

Temple Israel
Boston, Massachusetts
June 16, 1948

PREFACE

I AM VERY HAPPY, indeed, that the Temple Israel Institute
on Religion and Psychiatry held in Boston at the end of
October, 1947, should be recorded in the permanent form
which this book affords. In designing this two-day conference of religious leaders of New England and distinguished psychiatrists and psychoanalaysts, I had the hope
that the sanctuary and the laboratory might be mutually
helpful and that this pioneering venture might prove the
inspiration for many such Institutes throughout America.
The enthusiasm both of the religionists and the scientists
who participated in the discussions during the sessions of
this Institute is indeed a happy augury for future co-operation between religion and psychiatry.

The goal of both disciplines at their best is to lead us
to an inner serenity and an inner maturity that will make
us friends rather than enemies of justice and peace.

Many people, depressed and pessimistic, think that the
trouble is with the world while often the main trouble lies
within themselves, in their own unsolved conflicts, fears,
and hates. Men and women who are engaged in "a Civil
War" within themselves can never write a genuine peace
pact for society.

Not that anyone today can deny the real difficulties
and dangers of our age — inflation, possible depression,
group tensions, hunger at home and abroad, and above all
the threat of atomic destruction. Economic and social
democracy can solve many of these problems and man,
who has learned to tame his destructive and aggressive
impulses rather well within the smaller circles of the city,
state, and nation, can, I believe, create a world law and a
limited world government before it is too late.

At the very best, however, the tensions in our age will

continue to be unprecedentedly great. That is why we need more mature minds than ever before. Courage to master outer danger emerges from serene and not perturbed personalities. Modern psychology can help normal people to retain their equilibrium or to regain it, and prophetic religion can give them both cosmic assurance and a sense of spiritual purpose in life. Both the laboratory and the sanctuary are indispensable if we are to overcome our emotional and moral turbulence.

Why is it that we are so often immature? We all carry our infancy with us, our whole past histories, and many of us are still fighting the psychic battles of twenty or even sixty years ago. Every child while possessing many potential qualities of love and generosity is at the same time greedy, envious of his family rivals, afraid of his inevitable inner angers. Notice how these childish fears and moods reappear in adult form in the areas of economics and politics, all dressed up, of course, in acceptable garments of rationalization. So often we want greedily to take in and do not know how to share our values and goods. Or we hate our rivals or fear them; hence, the quite irrational battle at times between management and labor. Or, cloaking ourselves in the garments of self-righteousness, we look at other nations as the embodiment of total evil without realizing that we have carried over into our adult years many of our unsolved infantile hostilities which we then project onto other groups and peoples.

One absolute necessity of our age is for us to grow up psychologically. In order to do this we have to understand our own weaknesses and shortcomings and likewise to accept the weaknesses of our neighbors, other men and nations. We must understand that often we ask the impossible of life — too much love from everybody, too little frustration, or the attainment of absurd goals of power and prestige. The truth is that life is very hard and often defeating and there are no secure guarantees in this precarious human adventure.

As a religious teacher, I hope that religion, utilizing the newest discoveries of psychiatry, will aid immature men and women to achieve new depth and inner integration. Religion need not and must not abdicate in favor of psychiatry; but it certainly should utilize the basic principles of mental health that the scientists have discovered, helping to disseminate them to millions of confused Americans.

What are some of these principles? One important truth is that we human beings should always expect relative and not absolute achievement in whatever we do or feel. A second important principle is that genuine insight somehow is healing therapy. If we know what we are and what we need psychologically and religiously, then we shall be able to manage ourselves far more artistically. When we cease being a mystery to ourselves, carrying around an unknown enemy, as it were, in our bosom, we are on the road to inner maturity.

Religion will be making an enormous contribution to genuine brotherhood when it comes to emphasize the truth, which is ever more evident, that there are no sectarian labels to our fears and aspirations, that there is no essential difference between the basic anxieties, phobias, hopes, and hungers of a Christian, a Buddhist, a Jew. Every child goes through similar stages of development. All human beings seek security, status, serenity; are afraid or ashamed of their aggressions, passions, and inadequacies.

Religion, equipped with the new tools of psychological science, can help people everywhere to understand themselves deeply, to master their undesirable traits and to fashion characters of strength and integrity.

It can teach our age that if people hate themselves, suffer from a needlessly overburdened conscience, feel rejected and defeated, they will be tempted to build a society of hate and of war. They will try to escape from themselves into violence.

This volume on religion and psychiatry is concerned with the attainment of a new maturity by the men and women of our age. Maturity is achieved when a person accepts life as full of tension; when he does not torment himself with childish guilt feelings, but avoids tragic adult sins; when he knows how to postpone immediate pleasures for the sake of some long-term values; when he makes peace with the unarguable fact that he is not omnipotent, nor is anyone else on earth, but that all men must share each other's frailties and draw from each other's powers. Our generation must be inspired to search for that maturity which will manifest itself in the qualities of tenacity, dependability, co-operativeness and the inner drive to work and sacrifice for a nobler future for mankind.

Actually men and women today are hungering for a profound faith that will give them a sense of relatedness to the Divine Power at work in the world, a faith that will understand that if one human being is oppressed, then the whole building of mankind is insecure; they are hungering for a religion that is universal in its outlook, wanting every human being to have his house on the good earth, a shelter from the winds and storms of nature and human nature, with the windows of that house always open in love to the entire world, a religion that is so magnificently realistic that it demands that each person shall love his fellow human being, his brother with all his defects, just as he loves himself with his own defects, a religion that will teach all of us before it is too late that we are placed here on earth as equally valuable children of the Divine King.

JOSHUA LOTH LIEBMAN

Boston, Massachusetts
May, 1948

TABLE OF CONTENTS

by Lydia G. Dawes, member of the staff of Children's
Hospital, Boston, Massachusetts; member of the Boston
Psychoanalytic Society; visiting lecturer at the Smith College
School of Social Work, Northampton, Massachusetts.

by Paul E. Johnson, Professor of the Psychology of Religion
at Boston University; author of *Who Are You?* and
Psychology of Religion.

by F. Alexander Magoun, Associate Professor of Human
Relations at the Massachusetts Institute of Technology,
Cambridge, Massachusetts; engaged in a consulting practice
on human relations in industry as President of Human
Relations, Inc., of Boston; author of *Balanced Personality*
and *Courtship, Love and Marriage.*

by Joseph J. Michaels, Instructor in Psychiatry at the
Harvard Medical School; Associate Visiting Psychiatrist
at Beth Israel Hospital, Boston, Massachusetts; Consulting
Psychiatrist for the U. S. Veterans Administration in
Boston.

by Eric F. MacKenzie, Pastor of the Sacred Heart Parish,
Newton Centre, Massachusetts; Officialis of the Metropolitan
Tribunal of the Archdiocese of Boston; author of
The Delict of Heresy.

INTRODUCTION

THE QUESTION OF THE relationship between religion and psychiatry is one which is arousing more and more positive interest in the minds of both religionists and men of science. There is a discernible trend in psychiatric thinking today which has reacted against some of the negative expositions of religion as they were advanced by the early psychoanalytic pioneers. More and more it is becoming clear that both religion and psychiatry can and do complement one another. However, this present volume on religion and psychiatry does not enter into the deeper theoretical levels where psychiatry has challenged religion. The theological concepts of sin, guilt and man's Fall demand renewed exploration with the assistance of psychoanalytic insight. The whole problem of ethics is also being challenged by the newer psychiatric studies, as evidenced by two such works as Flugel's *Man, Morals and Society*, and Erich Fromm's recent *Man for Himself*. Both are attempts to reformulate man's ethical relationship to himself, to his fellow man and to God, and thus it is becoming increasingly clear that students of psychology are no longer content merely to observe but are delving into the entire field of values. In the realm of values, both religion and psychiatry must continue to deliberate and provide ample room for further re-evaluation.

As a record of the Temple Israel Institute on Religion and Psychiatry which was conceived by Dr. Liebman and sponsored by the Temple Israel Brotherhood, this volume attempts to deal with much of the pragmatic nature of psychiatry and is an introduction to many of the subtle insights discovered by the psychiatrist and the psychoanalyst. It grew out of the attempt to give clergymen who are aware of the necessity for newer techniques and profounder insights in their counseling work some of the observations made by scientists in the field of human relations. There is little of philosophy here. That must be reserved for future students. Rather, in this collection of pragmatic papers, the endeavor was made to acquaint the clergymen with the many ramifications of the growing field of psychiatry in the United States. Thus, in the paper presented by Dr. Harry Solomon we gain some insight into the work of the hospital as it attempts to treat psychiatric patients and afford them effective therapy. On the other hand, the symposium was fortunate in having secured the services of Albert Deutsch, columnist for the newspaper *PM* (now *New York Star*), who has inherited the mantle of Dorothea Dix and other crusaders for mental health in the United States. Mr. Deutsch presents a picture which might have been called "Inside U.S.A. — Mentally Speaking." He reveals some of the glaring defects and abuses in the mental institution and emphasizes the great responsibility which not only the doctor but society as a whole has in taking care of these patients who must of necessity be kept in isolation.

The main part of the symposium dealt with the structure of familial relationships as they were delineated by Drs. Gardner, Berezin, Dawes, Michaels and Magoun. The papers in this section are more or less descriptive of the problems within present-day family life and how they reflect upon the emotional (and religious) health of those involved in the human situation. The religionist should be careful to notice the great sense of compassion and profound sympathy which these scientists display for the patient and their growing awareness of social conditions as they influence the shaping of personality. In this regard, one may well wonder if not more than a kernel of truth was expressed by Dr. William H. Sheldon in his book, *Psychology and the Promethean Will*, when he said, "Psychoanalysis, for example, is far more a religious than a medi-

cal problem"; or, in another place, when he wrote, "Psychoanalysis is, then, indeed nothing more mysterious than a
highly specialized technique for dealing radically with des-
perate religious problems." In this sense, the scientific students have enriched greatly the religionist's perception of
the necessity for deeper understanding of the human pattern of growth. This appreciation is especially seen in the
section which deals with the problem of "Religion and
Psychology — Where They Meet and Part" as presented by
three outstanding clergymen, all of whom have had espe-
cial training in the psychiatric field. Their synthesis should
provide further common ground for future understanding
between the two fields.

It is to be hoped that symposia such as these will be
continued, as the interest shown during these meetings
sustained itself throughout two days of listening to the
many-sided papers which were presented.

This volume is indeed proof that religion and science
are no longer in conflict but recognize their interrelated-
ness, as science provides the techniques and religion the
values by which men must live and grow.

ALBERT A. GOLDMAN

PART ONE

WHERE PSYCHIATRY AND RELIGION
MEET AND PART

CHAPTER ONE

FIVE AREAS OF MUTUAL ENDEAVOR

Seward Hiltner

WHEN TWO PROFESSIONAL GROUPS come together there is a strong temptation to follow one of William James' classifications of temperament, that of the tender-minded and tough-minded. The tender-minded are likely to confine themselves to thinking up all the true and nice and cooperative and pleasant things about the other group, and then to say these things as gracefully as may be without flattery. The tough-minded, on the other hand, are impelled to use the occasion, with all courtesy and artistic skill — albeit devastatingly — to demonstrate to the other group the extent of its deficiencies.

The clear inference of the title, "Where Psychiatry and Religion Meet and Part," is that both tenderness and toughness should be checked at the door. Fortunately for me, such checking happens to be in accord with my views and feelings on the subject. And yet, though what I shall strive for is objectivity, it cannot be through a detachment which ignores the fact that I am a clergyman, not a psychiatrist, that I have biases and am not above either the wedding or the battle. The relative amounts of tenderness and toughness I have in my pockets are something about which my readers must judge.

Meetings happen in places. There seem to me to be five kinds of places at which psychiatry and religion now meet, and where, by implication, they will meet still more in the future than they have met in the past.

The first place where psychiatry and religion meet is what we may call, for short, "the clinic." The clinic may be

3

a hospital, a prison, a case-work agency, an out-patient service, or something else. It is an institution or agency or even a method of private psychiatric practice where professional therapeutic services are carried on under the administrative direction of professional groups other than the ordained representatives of religious institutions.

Hospitals are run by doctors, and their psychiatric services and wards, by psychiatrists. The psychiatrists are responsible for the total welfare and therapy of the patients in psychiatric wards. Anyone else on the staff – be he nurse, social worker, librarian, clergyman, or some other – touches upon the work for which the psychiatrist has final responsibility.

At such points we are witnessing an increasing meeting of psychiatry and religion. On the side of religion, there are today more chaplains in such clinical settings as hospitals than at any previous time, more clergy and theological students taking clinical pastoral training (which, among other things, prepares them for work in such a setting) and more attention is being given to the study of approach and methods in pastoral care and counseling.

On the side of psychiatry, there is less of what might be called therapeutic imperialism, and an increasing recognition of the capacity of others like the clergyman to be of help to people in a psychotherapeutic sense. Psychiatry began its modern career as a branch of medicine charged with the care of psychotic patients, those with serious mental illnesses. In the last century, like medicine itself, psychiatry looked only to physiology as being the "real" thing which would unlock both the causes of and treatment for mental disorders. But brilliant minds, and the painstaking application of clinical investigation, led it early in this century to consider psychology also as being "real"– and to see both the causes of disorders and the kind of therapy that could cure them as residing within the sphere of the psyche as well as the soma, in interpersonal relationships as well as in bodily interventions. The investigative methods of the natural sciences, properly translated, proved immensely fruitful in explaining how man *as man* operated, as well as in elucidating how man operated as a creature who digests, and cuts his finger, and gets an ulcer.

The further psychiatrists have explored, the more they have seen that even bodily diseases and accidents are seldom uninfluenced by the psyche of the patient—his attitude toward things, what he gets mad at, his secret ambitions, his half-recognized fears. At the same time, increasingly useful methods have been discovered for helping people whose difficulties are rooted in the psyche. The psychiatrist has learned a great deal. He is not exaggerating if he says his discoveries about cause and treatment have potentially doubled the range of medical knowledge and practice.

But the psychiatrist today is not a happy man, for he stands between two worlds — that of medicine and that of religion. He has the uncomfortable and not wholly welcome task of mediating between the physical and the spiritual. He must bethink himself sometimes that no man can serve two masters, and wonder if there is any real alternative to cleaving to one and despising the other. If he lets values in, he has the uncomfortable feeling that he is getting away from natural science. But if he tries to remain purely descriptive, his clinical conscience may prick him for omitting something vital.

To date, one of the main practical solutions of the psychiatrist's dilemma has been what could be called "administrative." He can supervise a clinic, for instance, and be "the therapist." But since he has a clinical eye and a concern for his patients, he can permit the social worker and psychologist and even the clergyman to assist in his work. He not only permits but welcomes them to his clinic or hospital or other center. So long as he is in charge, his medical colleagues will believe he is still a natural scientist unseduced by the world of values. On the other hand, when, on occasion, his social worker or chaplain establishes excellent rapport with one of his patients and does far more in helping toward solution or cure than he himself has been able to do, he has a difficult time if he attempts to maintain the fiction that there is a basic difference between what he does and what the others, in given circumstances, can do.

In another realm, as we shall see, the clergy have been victims of situations that have led them also to a kind of imperialism. But in the clinic it is the unsought imperialism of the psychiatrist that controls, and that, therefore, must be transcended if psychiatry and religion are to meet there as they should.

When the Protestant conference of clergy and psychiatrists met last winter in Washington, there were, at first, attempts by both groups to define their respective fields by what could be called "fence-building." That is, "Inside this boundary is my domain; you stay out." But this trial lasted only a few minutes, for it is manifestly not the right way to define these functions. The solution came with the suggestion that the clergyman and the psychiatrist each had his own more or less clearly defined *focus of function,* but that the overlapping and borderline territory was very broad indeed. Attention was then, and properly, diverted to a better understanding by each group of the focus of function of the other, that is, to its central standing point; significantly enough, the borderline areas then took care of themselves without the necessity for detailed legislation.

There is, I suspect, no generic instance of a type of malady to which one can point and say: That is only for the psychiatrist, or only for the clergyman. Even with help in bereavement, traditionally the field of the clergy, Dr. Erich Lindemann and his colleagues have shown how enormously important the services of the psychiatrist can be in some instances. In the field of help to psychotics, traditionally the exclusive stand of the psychiatrist, Dr. Anton T. Boisen and others have demonstrated that the clergyman can sometimes perform therapeutic service when the patient may be inaccessible to anyone else.

In the clinic — that is, in those places where therapeutic service is administered by psychiatrists — the clergy are vastly more welcome than they once were. When Dr. Karl A. Menninger was setting up the training programs for psychiatrists of the Veterans Administration at Winter Veterans Administration Hospital, one of his urgent concerns was to have on his staff chaplains who could interpret and demonstrate to psychiatrists-in-training what a clergyman can do working side by side with them. The clinical pastoral training programs are now welcomed in almost any hospital or psychiatric ward where psychiatrists are on their toes, and great progress has been made.

It is true that we clergy and chaplains, in such situations, must still very often work in a "fixed role" on the therapeutic team. We may be informed that therapy is performed by the psychiatrist; testing, by the psychologist; family contacts, by the social worker — and that our job is religious, with the implication that it is something quite different from therapy. We find such definition by fence-building to be a little behind the times, for we have seen, in a few places, the results that can come from a more "fluid role" type of therapeutic team. If the chaplain is able to make the best contact with the patient, then he will, in effect, be given the major therapeutic assignment with this person — even if it be not breathed above a whisper that what he is doing is therapeutic.

There are good reasons, indeed, why the psychiatrist

should have oversight and be general administrator of such clinical work. But the gradual replacement of the teacher-pupil relationship by the colleague relationship is bound to come. The present imperialism is understandable but unintentional. The clearer the view of the realities involved, the more rapidly will the real capacities of colleagues like the clergyman be recognized at their full value in the clinical setting.

The second place where religion and psychiatry meet is in those pre-therapeutic activities we call education for mental health or for peace of mind and spirit. The tremendous national response to Dr. Liebman's remarkable book, *Peace of Mind,* has demonstrated that people feel that the messages religion and psychiatry bring are very closely related, or ought to be.

Consider the notable concomitance of some contemporary developments. Pediatrics has moved far from being a mere matter of physiology, or of tracing children's ills to parents. No good pediatrician any longer ignores parents, but neither does he think that merely telling parents how to treat their children properly will accomplish the desired results. He needs to know how to change parents, not merely to know they ought to be changed. He has, in truth, become a psychiatrist not only for children but for parents as well.

Churches are increasingly awake to the fundamental needs of children: church nursery schools, week-day schools, vacation church schools and summer camps — all are laying increasing stress on building a program that recognizes the interests and needs of the children of different age groups, and that takes individual differences fully into account. Are not these two developments at least parallel?

Or consider the other end of the span of life. Just at the time when geriatrics is beginning to receive the serious attention it deserves (and there bids fair to be a specialty in medicine of that title) the development in the church is symbolized in the two-year Study of Religious Ministry to Older People now being carried out by the Federal Council of the Churches of Christ in America. Geriatricians, like pediatricians, are going to have to be psychiatrists as well as physicians. What older people think and feel will prove as important as what children think and feel. And, once one has conceded the importance of the patient's own frame of mind, one is bound to follow the course that is now so far along in the field of pediatrics. In our research on pastoral help to older people, we are not only incorporating into our methods whatever doctors and social workers and others are prepared to teach us; we are also using the best pastoral methods we know in helping specific older people, and are recording the results so that we can study objectively what is and is not of help.

The other night on a suburban train I met a psychiatric social worker — he might just as well have been a psychiatrist — and we discovered we were headed for adjacent towns in order to teach courses that sounded suspiciously alike. His course bore the title "Human Relations." In explaining it he said, "I'm really trying to talk about everyday problems of living, not about psychiatry or social work in any technical sense." I found myself saying, "My course is called 'Psychology,' and of course I'm trying to deal with understanding ourselves, and our resources for everyday living, rather than about psychology in any technical sense."

Perhaps the general recognition of the significance of the emotions and the feelings, which the psychiatrists have done so much to elucidate, has now become more general than we have realized. If we are to touch people where they live, and aid them in finding resources for the natural problems of everyday living and human development, it is inevitable that we both pay more attention to just that and — in the educational setting — pay less attention to whatever is purely professional, or technical, or even distinctive about our own focus of function. For as we concentrate on the need of our group, we find that the resources brought out to meet it are neither psychiatry nor religion nor social work nor anything else alone, but something bearing traces of them all.

The broader test of work performed is not alone what it does for individuals, but is what happens to the community. Psychiatrists began with psychotics, moved to a concern for psychoneurotics and thence to psychosomatic medicine: they broadened further to think of social and preventive psychiatry; and now are coming to think of the large social job of psychiatry as being much akin to the task of public health. With no diminution of interest in individual and small group therapy, they show increasing concern — within the limits of the attainable number of personnel and funds in sight — to spread their services so as to do the most good. There seems to be a probability that one county in New Jersey will soon appoint not a mental hospital superintendent, but a Director of Psychiatry for the whole county. Such moves for the extension of service are admirable.

Part of the test of whether either religion or psychiatry, or both, are doing their job well is to be found in how many mental disorders are being prevented, how many types of case work services can be expertly performed by available agencies, how much juvenile delinquency is nipped in the bud and the boys or girls helped to find useful outlets for their energies, how many vested interests of any kind are kept from exploiting the interests of all the people.

Neither the pastor nor the psychiatrist are full-time social reformers, nor are they politicians, except perhaps at ecclesiastical and psychiatric gatherings respectively. But both approach the problems of the community with special knowledge of man's needs and abilities, problems, frustrations, and potentialities. The church is an old hand at this community business, and sometimes, therefore, a bit too sure it knows what is good for the community, or else standoffish because the community seems to consider its standards as idealistic and impracticable. The psychiatric group sometimes tends to stand aside on its technical dignity; or, if it gets in, to go through a period of enthusiasm which, forgetting its own psychiatric principles, may easily turn later into rejection of the obligation.

The fourth place where religion and psychiatry meet is in the patient or parishioner himself. Let me try to illustrate what this fateful meeting now means, and can mean on an even larger scale in the future.

Psychiatry discovers, among other things, that patients who have little capacity for relatedness to other people also lack fundamental self-confidence and self-respect. They draw the conclusion, therefore, that preoccupation with one's own personality, far from being a confident interest in the real self, is far removed from self-respect. They conclude, in other words, as Erich Fromm has so ably demonstrated, that selfishness and self-love are not only not the same thing, but are poles apart.

The religions of the Jewish and Christian traditions, with their fundamental ethical interests, have also been concerned about man's preoccupation with his own apparent interests which conflicted with his relationships to his neighbor. Looking back, one finds more than one theologian who had at least a good measure of insight into the concomitance of response to the self and to others which psychiatry has recently clarified. But religion must also acknowledge that we have all fallen into moralistic patterns through failure to set forth this fundamental truth. If any significant attack is to be made on selfishness, an approach must first be made to the problem of building up self-respect.

Here we see a deep truth about man, sensed by religion through the ages, at least adumbrated by great minds of the church, but often pushed aside because the implications might be misunderstood in terms of renunciation of social obligation. Psychiatry has so clarified it that it cannot now be ignored. The parishioner who is preoccupied with his own concerns must be seen to be operating under compulsion; and no exhortations to him on his obligation to other people can possibly help him or his relation to other people unless preceded by a clarification of his attitude toward himself and an enhancement of his own self-respect. He cannot find the courage for a step until he knows he has something on which to stand. He is not free. As the functional task of religion is seen, in its psychological setting, as much more a task of liberating than of channeling, it will mean that this fundamental insight of the psychiatrists is being used.

On the other hand, further reflection indicates that there must be some reason why such a truth, paradoxical as it is, and sensed by so many great theologians, was not more clearly stated down through the ages. Perhaps there is a real danger that, in discovering that self-feeling and feeling for others are concomitants, and that the Golden Rule does not condemn self but puts others alongside self, people may be inclined to stop there. It is no criticism of psychiatry as such to point out that some former patients, while integrated and able to move under their own steam and have some relationships with other people and respect for themselves, nevertheless seem bound by the four walls of narrow interests, while the needs of the world obviously call for more than that. Inner release, as we would see it, is not a final point but a stage — an indispensable precondition, not an ultimate goal. This suggests inevitably that psychiatry, whether wanting it or not, must think of an ethics, if not of religion — unless it is clearly to confine itself to dealing only with aspects of the personality and not with the personality as a whole.

One psychiatrist has stated that few patients who come to him today have hesitation in launching out about questions of sex; that is, they assume he thinks sex important. But few discuss religion with him in early interviews because they assume he will not consider it important. Often, he adds, the real nub of the difficulty is reached only when the larger attitudes towards the universe and God come into the discussion.

So I believe the discussion about the connection between attitudes toward oneself and toward other people must be carried one step further. One can affirm God, or love God, or — to put it in neutral terms, come to grips with his own destiny as a human being — only in the degree that he can affirm or love his essential self and other people. Conversely, if he can genuinely worship and love God and affirm his own destiny under this universe in which we live, the inference is clear — that he has some degree of capacity for relatedness to other people and respect for his inherent self.

As a creature between two worlds, man's conception of his own destiny is as real and vital a fact of life as is his relatedness to himself or other people. Until he has found the best and, for him, the highest possible answer to this question, by so much he is lacking in wholeness. Neither religion nor psychiatry, alone, could have seen the full implications. Together, they can see that all three types of attitude are concomitant, and discover a vital relationship among them. They can also see that, whether help is given on relationship to God or relationship to the self, if well done, it lays the groundwork for transference of the gains to the other relationships.

Finally, psychiatry and religion meet in the church. For let it not be assumed that church and religion are the domain only of the professional religious leaders, or that the psychiatrist is not, at least potentially, a leader in the church as in his profession. Psychiatrists are a professional group; psychiatry is what they practice in helping people; but the church is not characterized either by being a profession or by the specific ways in which it goes about helping people — but first and foremost in its being a fellowship with certain common convictions and purposes.

Despite occasional excerpts from sermons of brother clergymen, I know of no concerted move to deny to psychiatrists membership in the human race, or any release from the needs and obligations and satisfactions of mutually supporting fellowship with other human beings in a context which looks toward a way of salvation for men and women who are lonely, anxious, driven, or in despair. Churches, being cluttered up with a lot of human beings, are not perfect; but psychiatrists, being accustomed to the mirages of perfectionism, can hardly expect an institution full of real people to be thoroughly purged before giving it their allegiance.

It seems to me that, more than formerly, psychiatry and religion come together in church. The unexamined anti-religious sophistication which infected so many men of science in the recent past is beginning to give way to something much more positive. One no longer has to renounce science in the eyes of his fellows if he goes to church.

But from this point on we have a dilemma somewhat like that which we described in relation to clinics. The psychiatrist is the "ordained" administrator of the clinic;

the clergyman, the appointed administrator of the church. If psychiatrists come to church, what does the administrator give them to do? Are they considered merely as laymen in the mass, whose service is to be only in terms of theological waiting on tables and ecclesiastical dish washing? Or is their expert interest, knowledge, and ability to be set to work on a level with its value? A psychiatric consultant to a church school might be a genuine aid. Or the insights of a psychiatrist might prove very valuable when confronting the human obstacles to a successful every-member canvass.

As church administrators, clergy are much tempted to take for themselves such positions and responsibilities as they consider important, just as the psychiatrist has done with therapy in the clinical setting. Unless this natural but thoughtless tendency is re-examined, we clergy may unintentionally prevent psychiatrists, even if they are in church, from performing their potentially effective service for the church.

As a fellowship, the church is not bounded by four walls; nor does service to the church consist only of those activities which take place under its roof. May it not, indeed, be that the church may be now in a clinic, now at a scout meeting, again in a market place, as well as before the altar? May it not be that a renewed sense of religious vocation as a call to meet human need, on the part of the clergy, may attract to a similar vocation and church allegiance the psychiatrists who are more our co-workers than many of them know?

As we have discussed the meeting of psychiatry and religion in the clinic, the centers of education, the community, the patient or parishioner, and the church, we have indicated that some meeting is inevitable at all these points, that the real questions are: On what basis?

Is the best basis understood? And what steps will improve the mutual advantage of such meetings?

In a measure, we have, therefore, also considered where psychiatry and religion part. For they part wherever meeting is potential but not actual — and that is more often than it ought to be. They part in the clinic when the psychiatrist reacts to an idea of a clergyman rather than to a flesh and blood pastor or when he fails to accept him as a colleague in the process of helping people who need help. They part in church when the clergyman returns this type of compliment. They part in education when the psychiatrist fails to recognize that his interest is touched unless it follows his traditional patterns, is called "mental health" or "emotional education"; or when the clergyman cannot see anything as religious if it fails to bear the label in billboard letters.

They part in the community when either has not troubled to get the requisite knowledge, or has fallen victim to standoffishness, overenthusiasm, or petulant disgust. They part in the patient or parishioner at any time they become interested in something different from his real needs, and acceptance of his ability, with a bit of help, to lead them to those needs.

Psychiatry and religion part too when they relinquish trying to understand each other. If a psychiatrist says conscience is often a doubtful asset, the clergyman ought to know what is meant and commend it, even though he may suggest sharpening up conscience so as not to imply nonconcern for ethics. If a clergyman says men must recognize their sinfulness before salvation is possible, the psychiatrist ought to know what this means, even though cautioning against identification of the fact of sin with a sense of guilt. The understanding needed is more than semantic, of course. To clergymen, the denominationalism of current psychiatry and psychoanalysis is as confusing as religious denominationalism is to many psychiatrists. Yet neither is without reason or value; and psychiatry, even as the churches, has under way something like an ecumenical movement.

If there can be present fundamental good will, and then honest examination and open mutual criticism, the benefits to human welfare may be very large. Though psychiatry and religion do part today, all too often, I believe it is a marital tiff, not a divorce. For they part only where there has been opportunity to meet. Honeyed words will not produce the fundamental good will which in turn can motivate further exploration. But honest examination, and appreciative attempts on the part of one to see the other's frame of reference and focus of function, can produce such study. And I am confident that the only possible result is more meeting and less parting.

CHAPTER TWO

IS THERE DANGER OF SUBSTITUTING PSYCHIATRY FOR RELIGION?

Otis F. Kelly

As HAS BEEN POINTED OUT, we should never forget that psychiatry is a special field within the medical profession. It is the specialty which deals with diseases which affect the mental functions. Those diseases are many and varied, and are very frequently caused by infections, injuries, and other purely physical causes. Many other of these diseases are caused by emotional stress and strain, beginning very often in infancy. Many psychiatric patients, especially children and juveniles, need treatment, but psychiatrists often discover that the treatment should be applied to the parents. That is a well-recognized fact — that it should often be applied to the parents and the teachers and other superiors.

The treatment of the psychoneuroses, I think, is of main interest, and, in order to treat psychoneuroses intelligently, it seems to me that we need some standard toward which we are aiming, and toward which the patient is or should be aiming.

Psychiatry is a relatively young science. I was graduated from medical school in 1920. While I was a student in medical school, the first course in psychiatry was introduced into the curriculum of Harvard Medical School, so that may give you an idea of how young the science of psychiatry is. One might think, from some of the things one hears and reads, that psychiatry was the oldest of the

18

sciences dealing with human nature and had already solved all of the problems of human nature. Needless to say, I don't think that it has.

But psychiatry, like any other field of activity that deals with human beings, must necessarily be based upon a concept of human nature; and a correct concept of what a human being is, where he came from, and what he is for, what the purpose of his existence is, must be found in psychology. It may also be found in supernatural revelation, but, before we accept the supernatural revelation, we should have a natural reason for our idea of the nature that is in us. And so we go to the science of psychology to get some clear conception of what we are dealing with when we deal with human beings.

At the risk of telling you something that you already know, I am going to try to outline very briefly our concept of what a human being is and the evidence upon which we base it. We could start with the axiom that the nature of anything is known from what it does. That's true in chemistry or any other science. And when we study man as man, we must take our evidence from what man does in which he differs from his fellow animals.

Admittedly, man is subject to all the laws of chemistry and physics, he is subject to all the laws of vegetative life; he is subject to all the laws of sentient life, including the emotions, which he shares with the other animals. But also, in addition to that, we see man performing actions which are not limited by space, not limited by length, breadth, and thickness, and not measurable in terms of material things.

To give you one example: The most spiritual of sciences is mathematics. By spiritual, of course, I mean dealing with that which is not limited by space. We begin to study mathematics with "one and one is two." One what? We can begin mathematics only because we have generated an idea which is not limited by space, which is outside of the material order.

In many other actions, of course — all abstract thinking, every time we determine our own course of action with our own will — we perform actions which are outside of the material order.

We are driven to the conclusion, therefore, that, while man is obviously a material thing, there must be something in his substance which is spiritual.

For many long centuries, in scholastic psychology, it has been taught that man is a composite of matter and spirit — matter and spirit united in such a way as to form one single substance. Modern psychiatry, with psychology following along in its wake, has rediscovered that man, in all of his conscious acts, is a single substance, and that, in order to treat the so-called mental ills of man, the psychiatrist or the physician or the clergyman must recognize all aspects of that substance. That is a very healthy rediscovery, and has been productive of probably more good than any other discovery of modern phychiatry.

About four hundred years ago, Descartes, by teaching that the human soul and the human body were two entirely independent substances existing and functioning independently, though united by the pineal gland (the exact function of which is unknown) started or gave rise to the so-called "mind-body" problem; and, for almost four hundred years, psychology has been plagued by the search for the nature of mind. In modern times, that search has led to the theory of the existence of several minds in each individual person, including the conscious, the unconscious, and the subconscious mind, speaking of them as though they were different minds.

The natural man is man as I have outlined to you. I think it is impossible to stop at that. I am going to bring in now supernatural revelation.

We know from revelation that man, in the beginning, was given something more than his natural powers, more than his natural status as a rational animal. God created him, I firmly believe, because he wanted a creature who could obey Him of his own free choice. All other creatures obey the laws that God made for them — the laws of gravity, chemistry, physics, vegetation, animal life, and so on. They all obey them; they can't do anything else. Man can, because, in order to make a creature who could freely obey Him, God had to give that creature the power to disobey Him. And, in the very beginning, man exercised that power — he disobeyed God. Why? The Scriptures tell us that Adam and Eve disobeyed God because the serpent came in. The serpent, from time immemorial, has been the symbol of wisdom. So, the wise man, pretending to be wise, disguised as a serpent, tempted our first parents, saying, "If you eat the fruit, you will be as gods" — you will be your own boss. And so they did, and they thereby fell from their elevated state of grace with a wounded nature, an injured intellect, and a weakened will.

Man was made to exercise his powers, particularly his specifically human powers, because the destiny of any creature is found in the exercise and the enjoyment of the fruit of the exercise of his natural powers. By the use of his natural powers, man can reason from effect to cause, and he can come to the knowledge of the Creator and does acknowledge Him as his Creator; he introduces disorder into his nature, into his general status, both natural and supernatural.

If you want to read a very accurate description of many of the present-day citizens of the world, go back to the first chapter of the Epistle to the Romans and read St. Paul's description of the pagans in his own day: "When they knew Him to be God and did not pay Him honor as God." He left them to themselves; God abandoned them to a reprobate, and, "thinking themselves to be wise, they became fools." And there are many psychiatrists and psychoneurotics today who think themselves to be wise but actually become fools.

⏤Where do psychiatry and religion meet on this subject? Both undertake to treat the whole man. The psychiatrist's job is to treat disease, whether it be of infectious origin, or traumatic origin, or emotional origin. There are mental conditions such as, to use one example, anxiety; the psychiatrist's job is to treat pathological anxiety. Pathological anxiety exists when a patient is very anxious and suffering from it when there is no adequate objective reason for that anxiety. But it seems to me that when a person is anxious because he knows perfectly well that he has done something contrary to the laws of God, and that he has gotten himself into a mess as far as his supernatural life is concerned, then it is the job of the priest or the clergyman to help him to re-establish his friendship with God; or, if his anxiety is based upon a certain notion about certain innocent things being sinful, then it is the job of the priest or clergyman to correct his error by proper instruction, because his anxiety is not a pathological anxiety when he is anxious as to the prospective results of his deliberate sin. It's perfectly legitimate anxiety — just as legitimate and healthy an anxiety as the anxiety of a man who finds himself unable financially to support his family, or something of that sort.

Unfortunately, the present-day situation in regard to certain conflicts between phychiatrists and clergymen, I think, falls into more or less the same category as the conflict which occurs between scientists in general and the clergy. In the clergy, as far as I know (I can only speak for the Catholic clergy) I see no conflict between science and religion. I see no conflict between psychiatry and religion. There is a great deal of conflict between scientists — some scientists — and religion, because some scientists refuse to see what is plain to their reason — namely, that there must be an intelligent Being Who made the laws that the scientists discover.

Some psychiatrists, I am sorry to say, having set themselves up to take the place of God, undertake to teach, sometimes, immorality to their patients. Three times within the last few months, I have asked to talk to the medical staffs of three different hospitals in order to inform them regarding certain points of morality as held by Catholic patients.

In one case, the doctor had been so ignorant of what the Catholics hold in regard to sexual morality that he had gone to the extent of asking the priest, the Catholic chaplain of the hospital, if he would reassure some of his Catholic patients because the doctor had advised them to masturbate and indulge in sexual intercourse freely — illegitimate intercourse. They were concerned because they thought such practice was against the teachings of their religion, and the doctor thought it would be nice if the priest would assure them that it would be all right. So, you see, not all the ignorance is on the part of the clergy, by any means. There is still a little bit existing in the psychiatrists.

I think that, by all means, the Catholic, Protestant, and Jewish clergymen should learn everything that they possibly can about human nature. Modern psychiatry has discovered many things regarding the memory. It has discovered that such a disease as schizophrenia, which used to be considered hopeless, is now, in some cases curable, and in many more cases capable of partial cure. When I started in psychiatry, if we made a diagnosis of schizophrenia and the patient later on recovered, we changed the diagnosis because we were so sure that it was a hopelessly incurable disease. And so there are other diseases. Manic depressive insanity — some one of these days, somebody is going to discover a chemical or physical cause for it — is still in the class with diseases like smallpox before the days of Pasteur. And so with many diseases; we just didn't know the causes of them, and every once in a while somebody discovers the cause of one. In the old textbooks about general paralysis of the insane, you could read column after column of the causes of general paralysis of the insane or softening of the brain. Now they have discovered the spirochaeta of syphilis filling the brains of such patients, and today these columns have disappeared from the textbooks, leaving one cause.

So I think there are a lot of the psychoses for which, some one of these days, we are going to find out the physical causes. In the meantime, psychoneuroses are definitely known to be caused by either intellectual error or emotional disorder. We should learn all we can about them and work with the psychiatrists.

But, if we believe what we represent, what we profess, we should not take the attitude that we have everything to learn from modern psychiatry. As a psychiatrist, I can assure you that the psychiatrists also have a lot to learn from religion.

I think the reason for the great enthusiasm today, outside of psychiatry and professional psychiatrists, for psychoanalysis, is that there is a tremendous percentage of our citizens who want to know the answers, especially when they reach adolescence and youth, and go to their clergyman for them and don't get them. They are under emotional stress, and the advertised place where they can get the answers now is the office of a psychoanalyst or some other modern form of psychiatrist. So we are the ones that have fallen down on the job.

There are a great many of these problems which are properly not the work of psychiatrists at all — clergymen should be the ones to solve them. Admittedly, one of the causes of failure, frustration, depression, and so forth, is the floundering around in life by people who have no final goal at which to aim. They don't know God; they don't know their natural destiny, much less their supernatural destiny—namely, to know, love, and serve God. They talk about God and they don't even know what they mean. Consequently they flutter from one goal to another, seeking satisfaction and distraction in pleasure, in business, in professional life, and other things, to the exclusion of the final aim of their life. On the rare occasions that they think, all they see at the end is death and nothing more.

I think that a goal in life is what we, as priests and ministers and rabbis, have to offer. As I know the large body of psychiatrists, they are honestly interested in their patients. They are honestly interested in what religion can do for them—not so much what the clergyman can do for the patient by becoming a social worker, or something of that sort (all of which is very good in its place), but what the clergyman can give them in the supernatural realm.

That's the proper part for the clergyman to play in the relationship between physician and clergyman, and I am sure that every physician (psychiatrist or no), is delighted to have the co-operation of the priest, or the minister, or the rabbi. We should seek to learn what psychiatrists have to teach about human beings, but we should be on guard against letting psychiatry become a substitute for religion, and there is great danger of that today. And if the clergymen don't get together and save the day, soon there will be no religion and there will be all psychiatry; the goal of life will be not God, but self-expression, the same goal that was held out to our first parents when the little wise old devil came up, disguised, saying, "If you eat the fruit, you will be as gods."

CHAPTER THREE

A CREATIVE PARTNERSHIP

Joshua Loth Liebman

BIBLICAL JUDAISM WAS PRIMARILY an intuitive awareness of the reality of God and the moral duties of man. Neither in the Five Books of Moses nor in the later Prophets do we find any syllogistic reasoning – any of the proofs for the existence of God such as we encounter in Medieval philosophy, Jewish or Christian. The early Biblical builders of Judaism, as Rabbi Solomon Goldman has indicated in his important work, *The Jew and the Universe,* were men most deeply concerned with associative living, with the good life on this earth. Prophets and Psalmists alike challenged mankind to seek peace – not a static peace but a growing, dynamic peace – of the individual within himself, in his relationships to his fellow men and to God. The inner serenity portrayed in our Bible is a great motivating power strengthening man to struggle for justice and righteousness upon the earth.

As the centuries passed, however, Jewish thinkers came under the influence of the giants in Greek philosophy and some of them sought to harmonize the revelations of God with the insights of reason. I need but mention Philo who wrestled with Plato, and Maimonides who wrestled with Aristotle, to indicate this trend in Post-Biblical Judaism. Medieval Christian Scholastics certainly shared profoundly in the attempt to assimilate many of the great insights of Aristotle into their religious philosophy. Today, when religious leaders seek to incorporate into their world outlook many new truths of reason – not merely of philosophy but of psychiatry as well — they are actually following in the path of a great tradition in Western theology.

It is obvious to all of us that ours is not an age of peace — either individual or social. It is an age where men and women are tormented and torn, riven with all kinds of inner conflicts. It is a world also menaced by the fruit of the "Tree of Knowledge," misused and poisoned in the social realm. As the two distinguished previous speakers have indicated, an era such as ours needs a creative partnership between religion and psychiatry, the sanctuary and the laboratory. Such a partnership can provide partial answers to basic human problems and can aid men and women blessed with new sanity and perspective to become architects of a more just and peaceful world.

Religion and psychiatry meet at one important juncture in their deep concern about the nature of man and his needs.

Throughout the ages man has been engaged in the quest immortally described by the Greek philosopher Heraclitus —"I sought for myself." The prophets of Israel, the saints of Christianity, a Maimonides and an Aquinas in the Middle Ages, have all been great pioneers in this eternal search for inner understanding. The discoveries of Shakespeare and Dostoevsky, to mention but two of the titans in the realm of literature, are still valid for us — discoveries about man's complex motives, his restless hate, guilt and love.

It was not, however, until Sigmund Freud arrived on the scene that humanity was given the brush with which to paint the detailed portrait of the mind. He has been the supreme cartographer of consciousness, the first scientist to draw a truly helpful map of the terrain of the psyche, to show future explorers where its hidden valley and its high peaks are to be found.

I am convinced that all of us in our century will continue to be indebted to Freud for his pioneering work in the nature of man, work that is constantly being revised, elaborated, and changed by the co-workers and successors of the master-psychologist of the ages.

What is man? Freud, in effect, proclaimed that man like all Gaul is divided into three parts — instinct, consciousness, and conscience. We are so complex and so difficult to handle just because our personality has to be built up out of a harmony of these three different phases of our nature, and the balance is so delicate, the scales so easily tipped in favor of our instincts or our over-punishing conscience. The human mind should be a little democracy with checks and balances between the three branches of our inner government — the realm of our instincts — the id — which provides the driving energies for life, our loves and angers and ambitions, — the realm of the ego — that part of the mind which is in contact with the external world and which enables us to judge reality correctly, and the third area — the super-ego or conscience built up out of the commandments and prohibitions of our first guides in life, father and mother or their substitutes. This division of man into three parts was not unknown to the scholastic philosophers and certainly not unknown to Aristotle or Plato. You might say that the modern psychiatrists' attempt to create a harmonious balance between these three phases of man's being is merely a continuation in the twentieth century of an age-old dream that Plato limned for us twenty-five hundred years ago. Inner harmony is the prerequisite of outer justice. When the different phases of the mind are out of balance, when one part plays the role of dictator, life indeed becomes miserable or tragic. Where the instincts rule, you have a delinquent; if the conscience is too harsh, too demanding with its load of guilt, unbearable and unborne, you have a neurotic.

The goal of man viewed from this standpoint, then, is a wise balance between his instincts, his intellect and his conscience — a small republic in which all phases of the whole person shall be given room for development. How wise in this connection was the interpretation of Fosdick of that great verse from the Psalms, "Bless the Lord, O my soul, and all that is within me, bless His holy name" . . . *all that is within me* — the passions and impulses sublimated and harnessed to the proper uses of reason and of goodness.

We all need to recognize, more than we do in our time, that we share a common human nature in spite of the uniqueness of our protoplasm and the differences in temperament and physique that Professor Sheldon has vividly pointed out in his recent volumes. I do not deny that each person is, in certain respects, unique. Our constitutions vary. Our life circumstances do profoundly modify our personalities; a child who has known security and love and a wonderful family atmosphere will grow up with an outlook upon life different from that of the boy from a broken home with all the scars of divorce and family bitterness, or that of the girl who, by the accident of death, was deprived of a father's love in infancy. The accidents of our personal history are, more often than we ourselves suspect, the real potters of our characters. A frightening operation, a long illness, the birth of a rival brother, the folly of an overprotective mother, the collapse of family fortune and security — all leave their scar tissue upon the membranes of our souls. Yet in spite of all deep biographical differences we do share a common human nature and are brothers under the skin emotionally.

Every human being, black, red, yellow or white, Catholic, Protestant, Buddhist or Jew, of whatever social status he may be, seeks love, fears rejection, yearns for understanding, feels guilt, experiences anxiety, and wants to feel himself a significant partner in the human adventure, a co-worker with God.

Psychiatry can be helpful in explaining to us some of

the psychological needs of man — the needs of each individual, in the first place, for a proper interpretation of life.

We still look at the world with childish eyes and see it often only as a place for our fulfilment or our frustration. The world is much more than that, but to many people it is emotionally either a nursery or a prison — a bottle of milk or a punishing ruler. The streets of life are full of men and women who look mature but feel miserable because unconsciously they want everyone to give them the milk of love, or fear that everyone will beat them with the rod of punishment. We falsify life that way because reality is usually neither so indulgent nor so stern as our parents once were.

A proper interpretation of life is indispensable for happiness because we are prone to misread and misunderstand what our parents wanted of us long ago — we took their frown, their word of disapproval, their gesture of disgust too literally. And as a result we have grown up with the unconscious conviction that sex is disgusting, anger is criminal, and life should be sweet and angelic. A little boy takes things very literally, and in the spectrum of his spirit there are but two colors, white and black, right and wrong, the permitted and the forbidden. He is a dualist, not a pluralist. It is only as we grow mature that we come to see the true spectrum of life with black shading off into grey and blue . . . and all the other hues of emotional reality. Maturity means that we learn how to read life correctly — to realize how often we have mistranslated the attitudes and moods of our parents — certain that there was hate or disapproval or shame there, when actually only guidance and firmness were intended. We do outgrow our childish awkwardness of body; let us outgrow our childish awkwardness of conscience.

Psychiatry can be enormously helpful to people just by indicating how widespread and common this misinterpretation of life really is. Actually there is great reassurance in the knowledge of the universality of our emotional problems and anxieties, our human aspirations and dreams. It is an aid to maturity to be told that we must not look upon the world either as a nursery or as a prison.

Another great psychological need of man is that of proper identification. Judaism, in presenting the stories of the patriarchs, the kings, the prophets, and the rabbis has made available hero-patterns to countless generations. Christianity in a somewhat different way has met the deep need on the part of its followers for great identification-figures. The story of these last tragic years in Europe with their incredible concentration camps is the story of men and women who retained sanity when they had some strong leader or some saintly martyr with whom to identify themselves . . . some hero in their midst, to give them the feeling that man is higher than the beasts of the field.

Actually, one of Freud's great emphases is that a person becomes what he is by imitating the world around him not only in childhood but all throughout life. If we have strong and courageous models to imitate, this is a source of blessing; unfortunately too often our models are themselves weak, frightened, and immature. One of the most liberating discoveries of modern psychiatry is that a person does not have to be bound forever to a neurotic mother or a cruel father; he can, sometimes only with expert help, obtain finer heroines and better father-figures with whom to identify. I think that we have to teach people in our churches and synagogues that they should not feel guilt as they often do if they throw off the chains of an unhealthy mother-love or father-domination and begin to achieve a relatedness to some greater hero-pattern, teacher, pastor, counselor, whoever it may be.

Another great psychological need of man is proper perspective. By proper perspective I mean the understanding that we are all scarred veterans and combat fatigue is our fate at one time or another in the battle of life. We think other pastures are greener — but that is just an optical illusion. All pastures of work and career and marriage are at times brown and bare but the foliage grows again.

Perspective is the wisdom to recognize that depression is the fate of every sensitively attuned organism like man. How should it be otherwise? We carry our whole past history with us and sometimes we feel the ache in our bones of old conflicts and childish expectations. *There is the squalling infant, the frightened kindergartner, the rebellious adolescent, dwelling in the mansion of precarious maturity.* Sometimes we advance and sometimes we regress. As Freud put it, we human beings are like a marching army — we leave troops of occupation to guard the captured country of childhood and adolescence but if the forces of maturity frighten us, seem overwhelming or invincible, we retreat to the territory we already occupied and entrench ourselves once again in the land of babyhood and puberty.

We must learn to take that retreat in our stride — to accept momentary moods of depression as normal. We are depressed for a thousand different reasons — because we feel guilty about a failure or an impulse or feel anxious about a plan or a pain. We human beings are living histories and unconsciously we sense the resonance of old fears and phobias. We never completely graduate from our emotional kindergartens.

Depression is the price we pay for our culture and our civilization; it is the price-tag of humanity. Do you think that man can go through all the vicissitudes of growing up from the stage of utter helplessness to one of relative independence, from complete self-centeredness to one of mature love — through all the mood-swings of suffering and triumph and still have the impassivity of stone or the thick shell of a turtle? Depression, from time to time, is normal for a creature with a cortex and a thin skin and tender nerves and the capacity to remember old hopes and to be torn with present ambitions and future dreams. Proper perspective means the achievement of a true tolerance for ourselves, with our angers and our abilities, an understanding that every person is progressive at moments and can express that hostility on the adult level without too great danger to one's self or to others, a recognition that there is really something likeable about us — incredible as that may seem to our overdemanding conscience—and that life is rich and fascinating just because it is made up of a thousand different temperaments and gifts. Let us not make ourselves miserable because we do not feel the way our neighbor does, for we must force neither him nor ourselves into the Procrustean bed of uniformity of feeling or of action. There are many equally valuable patterns of work and worth in the world.

Further, all of us are defeated in one way or another. Let us indeed accept our inner climate as variable . . . sometimes we live in the Arctic Circle and sometimes in the Tropics. Our emotional weather is made up of hurricanes and tornadoes and gay smiling days. . . . It is hard to remember the sun when the shutters blow and the wind rattles and roars. . . . "This too will pass away". . . the sun will smile again. . . .

Modern psychiatry helps many individuals to attain a new integration and maturity through the fulfilment of these basic needs: proper interpretation, identification, and perspective. When the scientists of the mind make available new resources for the good life upon this earth, they are at that moment great potential allies of prophetic religion. It is basic to my own Jewish tradition that God reveals himself anew in every generation and some of the channels of this revelation in our day are in the healing principles and insights of psychology and psychiatry.

Religion, however, certainly can and must do certain things quite beyond the scope of psychiatry. It presents man with the moral goals of life; it portrays the spiritual ends of our existence. Psychiatry, by its very nature as a therapeutic device, cannot hope to grapple with the profoundest issues of human destiny. The sanctuary and the laboratory can learn from one another and can be mutually helpful in taking broken disordered personalities and making them one, as God is one.

When I turn from the realm of psychiatry to religion, I speak necessarily out of my own Jewish background, as Father Kelley and Dr. Hiltner have spoken so eloquently out of their own religious traditions. In Judaism we find a concept of God, a faith in man, and an understanding of our human tasks and responsibilities which can be enormously helpful in the fashioning of the good life on earth. Now to the great Jews of the ages, God did not mean a heavenly grandfather sitting in the clouds, a literal king seated on a throne of sapphire. These descriptions of God are just metaphors and similes, never to be understood childishly or naively. What the sages of Israel meant by God was the Creative Power, Process and Mind in the universe. Not that they were ever unaware of the evils, injustices and sorrows of life. The Book of Job in our Bible immortally describes a man who out of his terrible personal suffering tried at first to deny and to defy God. Then, lo and behold! God speaks out of the whirlwind — the majestic Power of the Universe symbolically says to Job in effect, "Little man, you want to know Me, the Creative Mind of the Universe? You seek to deny Me, the Creative Power in all of life? Where were you, little mortal, when I fashioned the foundations of the earth, the morning stars that sang together, the depths of the sea, the heavenly treasures of snow, the east wind, the gentle rain, the mystery of birth?" Job grows humble, beginning to recognize what colossal arrogance it is for such a tiny flame as man to rebel against the great Sun.

It is not only in the Book of Job but in other great Jewish philosophers and thinkers that we discover many truths about God. Philo, the great Alexandrian Jewish thinker several thousand years ago wrote, "Just try to flee from water and air, from the sky or from the whole of the world. We are of necessity caught in their compass for no one can flee from the world; but if we cannot hide from parts of the world and from the world itself, how can we hide from the presence of God?" Or as the Zohar, the great source-book of Jewish mysticism expresses it, "There are gates in the world by which God is known"—gates of history, and of conscience, and of science. . . . While a full knowledge is beyond the reach of any human being, the Holy One, blessed be He, makes Himself known to each one of us according to the measure of His understanding. . . .

The atheist really is an idolator worshipping at the shrine of his own little mind. Confidentially he believes that he has all of the answers while his answers really are premature and partial. The true religionist from the time of Job to Philo to our own day is a seeker after God, sometimes tortured in that quest, sometimes tranquil, but never arrogant in his conviction that he has the final answer.

When he has become wise, he has refused to judge the novel of the universe by the little chapter or the small page that he is reading or writing in his own lifetime. He knows that much comes before, and much will come after him. He realizes that there is a great Pen, an infinite Mind at work, and he recalls the lesson of Job, that every morning we awaken to a universe not of our own making, a world of miracle, majesty and mystery, and though we shall never find God completely we can discover traces of His Being in the stars and the atom, in the snow and the rain and in our own minds. When we run from God, He is the carpet on which we flee; when we rebel against Him, it is with His weapons of reason and intellect that we revolt. The thoughts that we think and the ideals that we treasure are His witnesses. Throughout our lives, whether we know it or not, the best in us is seeking the Divine; it is that search that makes us human.

In the Jewish tradition I find not only creative insights into the meaning of Divinity but also a new hopefulness about humanity. A distinguished scholar in Judaism recently has recalled to us the vivid ancient parable — that God found his messengers in the most unlikely place — amidst the degraded Hebrew slaves of Egypt. What a sorry lot those slaves were in Pharaoh's time, and yet from those beaten men and women arose a new light for the world. This parable asserts that it is not what man is today, but what man can potentially become in the infinite tomorrow that is all-important. Man may not *be* good today, but he can *become* good through the spark of divinity within his nature.

Is this just a consoling fairy story? No, I think that this belief in the potential greatness of the human species is verified in every clinic and laboratory where men and women are released from their private Egypts of distortion and conflict. Just as God saw in those disunited and despondent Hebrew serfs in the Nile the seed of future prophets, saints and kings, so we human beings in our century should not condemn the present as the end of the human story but see in today with all of its tragedy and its evils the promise of tomorrow's Sinai.

Actually in Judaism there is a very realistic understanding of human nature as a battleground between "the good impulse" and "the evil impulse." There is also a profound optimism that even the evil impulse can be made to serve a life-affirming purpose, for as the rabbis point out without the driving energies of the emotions within man "no one would marry or beget a child or build a business." All of the varying aspects of man, including his competitiveness and rivalry and passions, can be harnessed to the chariot of goodness. It is my faith that we can sublimate and master the evil within us in the service of righteousness and of life.

Man is an imperfect creature; he is not destined to attain the absolute. Growth, not perfection, should be our goal. When we understand that we shall torment neither ourselves nor others; we shall be realistic and honest enough to admit that there are elements of hostility and aggression in every one of us, but that these can be mastered and transmuted into things of art and creations of love. Anatole France said a very wise thing when he asserted that only those who expect modest things from human nature will learn to be kind and tolerant. Those who expect too much and receive too little will end up by turning into misanthropes, fanatics, or tyrants.

All of us are capable of hating as well as loving because we experience not only fulfilment but frustration from earliest babyhood through adult life. A great function of religion is to create in us a love that is mature and without boundaries. Religion can teach us to subdue the hostility in the human heart and can make us deeply suspicious of the hate that becomes projected onto groups — Catholics in one part of the world, Protestants in another, and Jews in still another. For it is quite true that multitudes do project onto other people the strange or savage emotions within themselves. They are afraid or ashamed to admit resentment for a father or hostility for a mother or a brother so they escape from their own private emotions into "hate movements," thus conveniently avoiding recognition of hostility and guilt in their own souls. Religion today more than ever before has the obligation and the opportunity to make all of us sensitive about our hate-feelings, suspicious of all of them until we become mature enough to attain "a moral equivalent for hatred," an anger against disease, poverty, intolerance and war — a truly creative indignation against the genuine evils of life.

The kind of love which religion must seek to make real in life is made vividly clear in a remarkable passage from an ancient Hebrew manuscript. An old rabbi asks the question, "How can we love the Lord our God with all our heart and soul and might when we can never see God, the invisible spirit of the universe? We can love God best by loving His letters best. Just as a child learns the alphabet one letter at a time and then combines the letter into words and the words into sentences until at last he is able to read a book, so should we regard every human being as but one letter in the alphabet of God. The more letters we come to understand and to treasure, the more we can read the Book of God and love its Author."

That ancient rabbi teaches us that the true meaning of life is to be found in this test: "Man, do you by your cruelty or callousness blur the letters of God or even erase them, or do you by your compassion learn to treasure the letters of God, your fellow human beings?"

Religion when true to its prophetic heritage does treasure the letters of God by investing every man with dignity as a child of the Divine. Psychiatry at its best also seeks to polish and preserve the consonants of Divinity — men, women and children — by making these letters glow luminously with integration and maturity.

It is characteristic of prophetic religion that it emphasizes the Messianic dream — the hope of a world redeemed from evil and purged of iniquity and freed of all the barnacles of pain and disease, a world that will become one as God is one. How far we still are from that Messianic Kingdom! We who live in this twentieth century recognize that there are no absolute answers and only partial victories;

yet these victories are good omens of a nobler and freer future when the letters of God on earth will not be blurred but rather will be burnished with love and understanding. The laboratory and the sanctuary can become allies and creative partners in helping to bring a little nearer that age of the Divine, by learning to work together with mutual respect, mastering together the new secrets of nature and of human nature, laboring together in the words of an ancient Hebrew hope and prayer "for the blesing of all, the hurt of none, for the joy of all and the woe of none."

PART TWO

HOSPITAL CARE OF THE MENTALLY ILL

CHAPTER FOUR

THE ROAD TO SUCCESSFUL PSYCHOTHERAPY

Harry Solomon

WE ARE ALL INTERESTED in the matter of preventive psychiatry, as we like to speak of it, the prevention of disorders of personality. That, however, is a field which has not yet been very thoroughly cultivated. It is a field in which the clergy, the physician, the sociologist, the educator, all will work together to form that fine new world in which everyone is totally happy, where no one has any dissension or hatred, where aggressiveness is always under control. That, I fear, will occur only after many more Indian summers have come and gone.

The major goal that we are now thinking about, as the next step along the lines of mental health, is the correction of difficulties at an early phase — the type of work that is being done in the mental hygiene clinics. The Judge Baker Clinic is doing that type of work in counseling, and we, as doctors, see the patients when they manifest their first symptoms that are "disabling." This is corrective rather than preventive; it is correction after things have begun to loosen up a bit.

I believe our techniques are improving year by year, certainly, if not month by month. Nevertheless, in the lifetime of any of us, there will still be the major breakdowns which have not been affected by any preventive attempts and which, if they are not readily corrected, lead over to the really severe and serious mental disorders. These are the cases that either represent very severe psychoneurotic manifestations or, as we have expressed it, psychoses. They are the cases of mental illness, requiring, perhaps, for their proper care and treatment, hospitalization. It is with this group of individuals that I am now concerned.

A hospital for mental disorders should be a place where the best that is available in the way of treatment should be offered and afforded, and the first problem in any hospital is accuracy of diagnosis. It should be thoroughly equipped with all the modern means and modern methods of study of an individual.

Hospitals should be equipped to reveal, in the first place, any physical defect that may be existing in the patient. Such physical defects may be causative, as in the case of brain disease and encephalitis, brain tumor, damage to the brain from injury, trauma, or they may be merely contributory, that is, an emotional disturbance having been started, there occur the difficulties of nutrition, let us say, and there is further difficulty that comes along. These must be discovered and corrected in order that one does a normal and wholesome medical job.

After one has delineated the problem as he sees it and has taken what steps in the treatment of the physical man are indicated, there comes the treatment of the specific problem, namely, the mental disorder. There are, as a matter of fact, in this era of medical knowledge, several methods that are particularly the methods of psychiatry. They include, first and foremost (perhaps the most important), the psychotherapeutic approach.

It is very difficult to define what we mean by psychotherapy. It is very hard to draw the jurisdictional boundaries between the activities of various people who deal with human beings. Psychotherapy, from the physician's standpoint, may be somewhat different than psychotherapy from the standpoint of others. Certainly, any relationship that exists between one person and another and beneficially affects the situation, is something that is extremely worthwhile. Whether that in itself is actually psychotherapy, there may be some question and some doubt.

Let me be a little bit specific: Suppose the gentleman on my left or right happens to be in trouble and comes in and says, "How-de-do" to me, and I pat him on the shoulder, and since I am a doctor, he goes away feeling better —"The doctor has done a wonderful thing for me." Is that psychotherapy? It is only psychotherapy if it is a situation that was thought out, that arose out of a knowledge of the basic underlying psychological mechanisms, that was applied with a distinct, definite purpose and can be re-applied to a great many people under similar circumstances with the belief that it will again be effective. In other words, psychotherapy must arise out of a knowledge of acquired psychological data; it must be something that is definitely directed for the benefit and the cure, for the healing or the help of an individual; it must be controlled, and it must be capable of repeated use.

So that our predilection with this matter of the treatment of individuals by psychological means (by interpersonal communication, by the relation of one individual with another) is something that requires a great deal of time and thought.

Whether we, as doctors or psychiatrists, are able to do this more successfully or less successfully than another group of individuals is hardly the subject of discussion. It is a fact that this is one of our tools, that it is a tool with which we as psychiatrists are particularly involved and with which we have been experimenting for years, trying to understand, to perfect, and to be able to apply in a specific way.

In addition to this primary psychiatric tool, we have a considerable number of individuals who are, as I said in speaking of diagnosis, suffering from an organic physical disease of the brain. It is our particular requirement to be able to take care of those individuals.

For example, for the last several years, we have been particularly involved in the treatment of syphilis of the nervous system with penicillin, a new modality in the treatment of human ailments.

There are, of course, a great many other diseases which affect the nervous system. I mentioned brain tumor; I could mention diseases of the blood such as pernicious anemia and many others.

The utilization of the knowledge of physical medicine, as it is applied to all ills of mankind, is another one of the tools that the psychiatric institution must utilize at all times.

In the last number of years there have entered the so-called "shock therapies," which have a certain specific place in the treatment of mental disorders. Among these is the convulsive shock produced by the injection of a drug into the blood stream or the application of an electric current to the skull, and thence through to the brain. This so-called "electric shock" treatment has an extraordinarily specific effect on certain cases of severe mental disorder. The majority of deeply depressed individuals can be returned to a state of pre-existing comfort, as a rule, in four or more weeks with half a dozen or ten applications of this method.

Another method is insulin shock, a rather complicated procedure in which, by the injection of large quantities of insulin, the patient is thrown into a state of very deep coma, allowed to remain in that state for an hour, and brought out with sugar; the procedure is repeated fifty or sixty times, day after day. This, again, has an extraordinary effect on a certain group of patients.

With these and other drug procedures, there have been made possible two things: (1) the improvement of disorders called psychoses; and (2) without completely eliminating the psychotic state, the patient may be brought to a condition in which the relationship of doctor, patient and hospital personnel may flourish. In other words a condition is attained in which psychotherapy can be applied.

In the use of these modalities good judgment must be used as to when and how they are to be applied. If, in most of the cases, one gets rather dramatic, successful improvement, one is still left with the problem of the needs of the patient who broke down because something had gone wrong in his life; while the symptoms have improved, the question is whether he will remain well without definite and specific treatment toward his personal problems.

With the use of some of these modalities which greatly shorten the course of an illness, it may be thought that we have lessened the work of the people who are responsible for the welfare of the patients. I think, on the contrary, we have increased it because we have placed more people into the community rather than leaving them in the hospital at a time when they need a great deal more help than would have been demanded had they remained chronically ill in the hospital.

Despite these methods that I have mentioned, there are certain failures; there are certain patients who go into the chronic condition requiring care. In the last ten years, another modality of treatment has been developed, namely, an operation on the brain for certain of the chronic cases, called lobotomy. This is a procedure in which the anterior portion of the hemispheres of the brain is disconnected by surgical cut from the rest of the brain. Curiously enough, some astoundingly good effects are obtained. Again, these people need care, re-education, retraining, and a variety of other things.

At the Boston Psychopathic Hospital, with our modern hospital equipment and setup, and with the methods that I have mentioned, our results in the early treatment of severe breakdowns are as good as in any other branch of medicine. Somewhere between 75 and 90 per cent of the patients that come to our hospital sick enough to require commitment return home greatly alleviated within six months to a year. I am dealing, as I said, with patients who were sick enough, distressed enough, and unclear enough to require commitment.

Not all the patients remain well. Some relapse. Then our problem is to go further and take care of the relapse. But it is a hopeful and helpful thought that the majority of the severely ill mental patients in the early period of their disorders can be helped and can be brought back into a very good state of adjustment.

Because of the good results of treatment in the incipient period of mental illness early recognition is of great importance. It is necessary therefore that the psychologist, the clergyman and the social worker be so well versed in the problems of mental disorder that they may understand the implications of symptoms. Certainly they should be aware of the probabilities of suicide in a distressed patient.

I will also add that it is necessary to have good diagnostic survey of people in distress because on the assessment of the prognosis, or what is likely to happen, as well as what must be done so much of the happiness of others depends. I need not say much about the necessity of recognizing the people with bad conduct who are often termed psychopathic personalities. They can do much damage to the kindly-intentioned counselor, clergyman, doctor, their families. Why should one assume a Pollyanna optimism in efforts that have no possibility of succeeding? This is what one does if one takes an unrealistic attitude and thereby fails to recognize the seriousness of the distortion of the personality.

With the patient in a hospital, we have, I believe, to

consider something more. Assuming an adequate staff of doctors, nurses, occupational therapists, psychologists, social workers, chaplains and recreation workers, good medical care will result. But there is a little more needed than adequate medical treatment. These patients are distressed human beings. Human beings that are not too distressed — you and I — have a great many difficulties to contend with in our everyday life. These are multiplied greatly in the seriously distressed and emotionally ill, and so we set down for ourselves the dictum that our problem is the twenty-four hour a day care of the patient rather than the few minutes, whether they be thirty or sixty a day, given by the doctor to the patient.

Our problem in addition to the specific medical treatments includes the type of care in which an individual, as a sensitive human being, can thrive. How are we going to accomplish that? First and foremost, of course, is the general atmosphere. The creation of a salutary atmosphere, in a hospital that is dealing with very distraught, sometimes noisy, sometimes destructive, frequently insulting individuals, is a matter of primary importance. Esthetics unquestionably help a lot. People are very much more well-behaved and get along better together in a nice room than they do in a very unpleasant one, and therefore the conditions under which individuals may live together are important.

In addition there are other facilities that one can make available under proper direction, including occupational therapy devices, physiotherapy, including tonic baths, massage, exercise and recreation. We must give the patient a sense of belonging and an ability to socialize with his neighbor.

This, then, is another of our great problems. How can we arrange for that situation — the situation of socializing the patient, of getting him interested, of again bringing forth his desire to be a member of society, to join with others, to have the pleasure of intermingling, intercommunicating with his friends, with those about him, with his family? All the things that I have spoken about play a large role — occupational therapy, physiotherapy, the medical treatments, nursing attention, and all those things. They put the patient into a particular sphere in which he is the center of attention, which, in itself, may do something to help him very greatly. However, in no hospital, as hospitals exist today, are they likely to be, except in the case of the very wealthy institutions where they charge a great deal, and even there, at times, they are often worse than some of our free institutions in socializing and supplying these needs.

In our public institutions, then, it is unlikely that there will ever be enough money made available to do this from a professional, paying basis. Perhaps that, in itself, is an advantage because we bring ourselves into the picture by having demands made on us to supply something. That has come about in several ways, particularly through students who are certainly not paid professionals. Students in a hospital are usually divided up into a number of categories. There are medical students, psychological students, clinical psychologists, social worker students, or occupational therapy students, and there are certain project students from our more modern types of colleges who come and work in the hospital for the purpose of serving the patients. In addition to these people, we have also had the Grey Ladies of the Red Cross and Women's Auxiliaries. In one hospital, the Boston Psychopathic Hospital, this has proved useful. It has been applied to other hospitals where budgets are strained.

With the admission of this type of personnel into an institution, one brings in a breath of the great outdoors, of the great outside world for socializing the patients, and it is much better than those of us who have our noses in the books and carry on our occupation day after day, year after year, until we think we know all about patients, and patients feel that perhaps we don't know about some of their problems. The ability to talk with the fascinated and perhaps fascinating young man or young woman from the outside who is devoted, in the first place, to learning and, in the second place, to serving, does an enormous amount to create an atmosphere in which the patient has an opportunity to thrive.

Under those circumstances, as I have said, the majority of our patients do thrive, and the majority of our patients are ready to go home. They are ready to go home from the standpoint that, in the hospital, they are doing very well; they are over their major difficulties; they are able to get along with their fellow man. They are ready, then, to go back into this terrifying competitive world in which they became ill; they have got to go back to the job which, perhaps, they have hated for a good many years. They have to go back to a wife or a husband who has been a nagger. They have to go back and face an economic situation that is very difficult. They have, perhaps, to take care of children twenty-four hours a day, which is something of a task.

Our next job, then, is the preparation of the individual for his return home and the preparation, as far as it is possible, of the home for the reception of the individual.

During the course of the patient's stay in the hospital, we have become acquainted with the family, and we know that very often the family members are much sicker than our patients. Certainly, they are very much more difficult for us to get along with, but they are able to tell us a few things that the patient is not able to tell. At any rate, we are acquainted with them, and our problem is to try to prepare the situation at home so that the patient will thrive. That is one of the places, certainly, where our skilled, experienced, trained, psychiatric social worker comes into the picture, and she has been in the picture from the outset of our system now in mode.

In the past, perhaps more than in the present, some of us used the church, the clergyman, more than we do today. The reason for that is that we now have much more able social agencies which will give us help, whereas, twenty and twenty-five years ago, it was chiefly the clergy to whom we could turn for socializing and re-establishing the patient.

The fact that these patients of ours will return in due course to their home is still a problem; they will return, we hope, to their original church; they will again be drawn into the family circle; the doctor, the clergyman, the social worker, and the psychologist, we hope, will all be involved in the continuing treatment of these patients.

At the Boston Psychopathic Hospital we have made a new step in this direction. Not all, but a very large number of our patients, when they leave the hospital bed, do not leave the hospital care. In fact, for some who are not too well as yet, we are beginning to have day care, so that they can spend the whole day with us and only have to meet the cruel world for fifteen, sixteen, or seventeen hours, during the large part of which they sleep, rather than the entire twenty-four. The others, the majority, come back to our institution for continuing psychotherapy, and, as I have already indicated, it is at this point that the social worker in our setup has a good deal of responsibility for the return of these patients to a beneficent and satisfying community.

Theoretically, during the period of hospitalization, when, as I have said, the doctor is thinking of the home situation, and the social worker is thinking of it, we have not in the recent past utilized the services of the clergy within our hospital walls, as we might well do in the future. In a few places in the world, this has been done, perhaps, but, by and large, it is an untouched field.

In conclusion, then, I should like to emphasize that, at the present period of our history, those patients who escape from the beneficent efforts or beneficent care in the early stages of their development and who go into a deep, growing psychosis (mental derangement) have an excellent probability, close to 90 per cent, that within a few weeks or a few months they will be back once more on the beam which will direct them toward outside living and a happy and satisfactory function. This state of hope and hopefulness means not less care from the standpoint of psychological adjustment, but rather more; because, as I said before, rather than staying as chronic hospital patients, it will mean that many of them will need to go home and require, perhaps, a maximum amount of care for some months until complete integration with society has taken place.

CHAPTER FIVE

THE ETHICAL STAKE IN
MENTAL HOSPITALS

Albert Deutsch

I THINK THAT OUR CIVILIZATION received, just a few months ago, a grave challenge to its own sense of decency and dignity when Dr. Karl Brandt, who was Hitler's physician in charge of the euthanasia program, instituted in 1939, testified before the American Military Tribunal at Nuremberg at the war crime trials. Dr. Brandt, in the course of his testimony, admitted that 275,000 German "lunatics" and other "cripples" were exterminated by the Nazi euthanasia program in the six months of its operation. In self-defense, he said that it cost the German government something like 25,000,000 marks a year to maintain its insane asylums and that a country could buy a battleship with those 25,000,000 marks. He said further that to continue the life of an insane person does not comport with the dignity of a state, and therefore it was a matter of state right to exterminate the insane.

When that news item was printed here (that was in February, 1947 and Dr. Brandt has been hanged since) I imagine there were a lot of Americans who felt horribly shocked that human beings could be coldly exterminated because of the fact that they were sick. And yet I wonder if we Americans have the right to distinguish ourselves in kind, although we can in degree, from what the Nazis did to their insane. We are not like the Nazis; we do not kill the mentally sick deliberately — we kill them by neglect, and I have some proof with me, culled from newspapers.

Just about the time that Dr. Brandt was making his defense at the Nuremberg court, an epidemic swept the state mental hospitals of Massachusetts and Rhode Island. Some 2,200 patients were stricken with this epidemic which, I think, was immediately diagnosed as intestinal flu. Its diagnosis was social neglect, and upwards of sixty of those patients died. I'd like to quote some of the statements of the institutional heads that were made at that time:

Dr. Clifton G. Perkins, Massachusetts State Mental Health Commissioner, said, "It takes the dynamite we have been sitting on to realize the seriousness of the shortage." Dr. John F. Hogan, Superintendent of the Rhode Island State Hospital in Providence, where twenty patients of the 500 stricken with this disease died, said, "The epidemic got out of hand in the early stages simply because we didn't have enough doctors, nurses, and trained attendants." The chaplain of that hospital, the Reverend L. L. Aber, said, "I blame the tragedy mainly on the failure of the legislature to appropriate adequate funds for maintaining this mental hospital. There are only thirty-one attendants here to take care of thirty-seven wards, and the base pay for attendants is seventy dollars a month for a sixty-nine-hour week."

Last week, the second of two patients was clubbed to death at the Fairfield State Hospital in Connecticut by another patient. Coroners are pretty hard-boiled fellows (a newspaperman learns that fact very readily) and I think that the statement made by Theodore Steiber, coroner for Fairfield County is quite significant. He said, according to a UP dispatch from which I quote, "Aroused public opinion is necessary to get some decent results at Fairfield State Hospital. At the time of the attack, in which this patient was beaten to death, the coroner said that there were sixty-seven patients in a single ward in charge of a 'timid little girl about twenty years old who was neither mentally nor physically equipped to cope with the situation.' Steiber said, 'The hospital has been in a precarious state for many years,' as he had pointed out in great detail in previous killings at the same institution."

In Cleveland State Hospital, in Ohio, about four months ago, three patients were scalded to death by another patient in an overcrowded ward that was in the charge of a former mental patient turned attendant. There was a big hullabaloo, as there always is in such situations, in the local press, about "Why isn't there an inquiry into Cleveland State Hospital? What's going on there anyway?"

In this instance, the superintendent of the hospital, Dr. Crawfis — one of the few mental hospital heads who will not permit himself to be made into a scapegoat — issued a public statement in which he said, "The real blame lies with the people of Ohio who have not given us enough to run the hospital properly." He alluded to the fact that the attendant was not qualified, as he was an ex-patient. "We have had to go out with clubs and beat qualified people into submission before they will take jobs paying eighty-five to ninety dollars a month."

Recently I received in the mail a clipping taken from the local Phoenix paper by the editor of my paper, *PM*, who has been vacationing in Arizona. This headline says: "Use of cuffs in hospital up to Chief." Then it says further: "Arizona State Hospital Board of Control members yesterday agreed that the use of steel handcuffs for violent patients be left up to the discretion of the Superintendent, thus ending a subject that has been up for discussion through the last three monthly meetings of the group." You can see how wisely this issue was settled. And it turns out that patients in a disturbed ward at this Arizona State Hospital are handcuffed with steel bands for days and weeks on end because there aren't enough attendants at this hospital to supervise the ward properly.

How civilized a people are we, really, when a headline like this appears, and a decision like this is made calmly by a group of representative citizens — that steel handcuffs for sick people are O.K. if the Superintendent, a harassed man himself, says the are?

A couple of years ago, Dr. Eduard Lindeman, then professor of philosophy at the New York School of Social Work, returned from a tour of the British occupied zone in Germany, where he had been giving orientation talks to the British soldiers. He told me that he had visited, among other places, the village and concentration camp at Bergen-Belsen two or three weeks after the British had occupied the town of Belsen, and he said, "The odor of burning flesh still hung over the village." You may recall that when the British took over the concentration camp at Belsen, 30,000 of its inmates were so far deteriorated that not all of the aid of the British liberators could prevent their deaths, and they died within three weeks after the occupational liberation.

Dr. Lindeman, who is a curious sociologist, went among the townspeople of Belsen, and asked them, "How do you feel about what happened at Belsen?" You remember that hundreds of thousands of people, men, women, and children, were belt-lined through the crematoria at Belsen, and Lindeman asked them, "What do you think of that?" And these townspeople shrugged their shoulders—"We didn't know what was going on there." The concentration camp was only a stone's throw from the village. He asked, "Don't you feel any sense of responsibility or guilt for what took place at Belsen concentration camp?" They said, unanimously, "Why should we feel guilty? We didn't do it. They did it."

That sounds pretty cruel, but I wonder again, on the

basis of my own inquiry into state hospitals, whether we can distinguish ourselves from them. I deliberately left out the south and the southwest from my tour, because I knew what I would find there, and I knew that if I played that up in my paper, people would shrug their shoulders and say, "What do you expect of the South? What do you expect of the backwoods of this country?"

I wish I could have taken you through Male Building A at the Philadelphia State Hospital, commonly called "Byberry," a little more than a year ago, so that you could have seen, as I saw, three hundred men, completely naked, in all stages of physical and mental deterioration, herded into a ward intended for eighty; and then have taken you through the piggeries on the grounds to see those carefully swept piggeries, and compare that neatness with the treatment accorded humans, three hundred human beings, by the City of Brotherly Love. I know that all of you would have had the same reaction as I did when I saw patients at the Philadelphia State Hospital eat their dish of macaroni and beets with their bare hands because there weren't enough spoons in that ward to eat with. Two hundred yards away from this place where six thousand patients were herded into an institution originally intended for thirty-six hundred stands the birthplace of Dr. Benjamin Rush, the founder of American psychiatry, the first psychiatrist at the Pennsylvania Hospital. That is the city where, two hundred years ago, Benjamin Franklin and a group of Quaker friends built the Pennsylvania General Hospital, not only for the physically sick, but for the mentally sick with the idea of restoring them, as I think they put it, "to recovery and the ability to earn livings for themselves and their families as soon as possible."

Today we talk about including psychiatric wards in general hospitals as if that were something new, when the first general hospital in this country specifically stated in

its charter that it was intended for the physically and
mentally sick alike.

In 1944, a grand jury of Cuyahoga County (in which
Cleveland lies) with the Reverend D. R. Sharpe as fore-
man, made a pretty thorough investigation of several
deaths of mysterious origin at the Cleveland State Hospital. The report of this grand jury, is, I think, unique in
this country, because it indicted no single superintendent,
no group of attendants, no group of doctors, but the whole
community of Cleveland.

I should like to quote part of that amazing indictment.
"The grand jury is shaken beyond words that a so-called
civilized society would allow fellow human beings to be
mistreated as they are at the Cleveland State Hospital. No
community dares tolerate the conditions that exist there. It
would be a prison for the well — it is a hell for the sick.

"We indict the civilized social system which, in the first
instance, has enabled such an intolerable and barbaric
practice to fasten itself upon the people, and which, in
the second instance, permits it to continue.

"We indict all who have abetted or even tolerated such
foul treatment of these unfortunate mentally ill, even as
history will indict us if we fail to redress this ancient and
inexcusable wrong."

That was in 1944. There had been very little change at
the time I visited it in 1946.

I won't go into detail on what I saw at Cleveland State
Hospital in 1946, except to say that in 1947 three patients
were scalded to death there; the Superintendent again told
the community that it was responsible, not he.

I hadn't intended to go down below the Mason-Dixon
line, but one evening I gave a talk to the Atlanta Mental
Hygiene Association, and I was pressured into attempting
a visit to the Milledgeville State Hospital. In all of these
visits to the mental hospitals which I wrote about, I had

my photographer accompany me and take pictures. And
so they said, "Let's have a picture, a documented story,
of Milledgeville Hospital."

Milledgeville is about sixty miles from Atlanta. There
were 9,000 patients there. This mental hospital was the
largest hospital in the world in terms of patient population. The Atlanta Mental Hygiene Association said, "There
are 9,000 patients down there, and we'd like to get something started." I said, "I hadn't planned to do anything
about the south," but they said, "Why don't you come
down?"

I called up Governor Ellis Arnall, and asked for permission to inspect Milledgeville. My paper, which is a liberal paper, had been vociferous in its support of Ellis Arnall
as a liberal governor. But Governor Arnall, to my surprise,
hemmed and hawed and said he would have to consult
every one of the State Public Welfare Board — he was only
governor, and the institution was democratically controlled
and he could not give me permission without the permission of the whole Board of Trustees.

I sent a wire back to the Mental Hygiene Association
— "Governor Arnall delayed giving me permission to go
down." They raised a fuss in the local press. I think it
is very significant that the trepidation of a liberal can
bounce back at him. To the amazement of everybody, when
the news got into the press that Governor Arnall was stall-
ing on letting me go into Milledgeville with a photographer,
who came to my defense but the late Eugene Talmadge!
Eugene Talmadge had been elected governor. (This was in
1946, and in November, the month previous, he had been
elected governor of Georgia; he died before January 15,
when he would have taken office, and there was a great deal
of trouble down there.) But, the week after that got into
the press there was a big lead editorial in "The Statesman,"
a paper run by Talmadge "What Is Governor Arnall

Trying to Hide?" and it hinted at Governor Arnall's terror about letting an "unbiased" newspaperman come and look into the murder of patients at Milledgeville. The next week, he followed it up with another blast at Arnall. The third week, I got a call from the State Public Welfare Director, inviting me to come down. This man, Judge Hartley, actually served as my photographer on that trip, and took pretty good pictures.

But I am not going into details about Georgia. I will say simply that it would require the eloquence of a Dante to describe adequately the hell that the Negro patients, particularly, of that institution underwent. I remember, when evening fell we were going through the building for Negroes, far in the back of the institution. We went into a women's building and there was no light whatever in some wards — and we had to grope our way from ward to ward. We would see these patients sleeping on bare floors, or on filthy, bug-ridden pallets that had been laid down on the floor, sprawled all over the place, even under the staircases. We had a flashlight with us, but when we lost the fellow with the flashlight, we wandered off. A couple of us wandered into what we thought was a ward; we didn't find out that we were in a lavatory until the women started to scream.

Let me tell you lastly about my own city. In New York, we have the greatest concentration of psychiatric resources in the whole country, if not the world.

We have 400 of today's 4,000 trained psychiatrists centered in New York. We have a lot of schools there, a lot of institutions; but I wish you could have accompanied me, less than a year ago, to Ward N-7 at Bellevue Psychiatric Hospital (which enjoys a world-wide reputation) and could have seen that crowded ward of women, one out of every four of whom was encased in a strait-jacket. This was in the fall, but I was told by the psychiatrist on the ward that summer presented a terrible problem. They had windows which looked very good and very modern, but which were impossible to open to let in air. In summer, the place was all heated up and there was no ventilation in the ward. It is charged that patients in strait-jackets actually died of dehydration in this ward. The few nurses tried to prevent fatal dehydration. "Every once in a while," one of them said, "we would pour a pail of cold water on the strait-jacket to cool it off."

This Ward, N-7, was the ward where, not long ago, one woman patient strangled another woman patient in a hydrotherapy room which hadn't been used for hydrotherapy for years. Four beds had been crowded into that room with no nurse or supervisor, and a patient got up and strangled another patient. Six months later, the same thing occurred in that ward.

We had, for six years, in New York, a beautiful eight-story building, the Kings County Psychiatric Hospital, in Brooklyn. It was unoccupied because the poor pay made it impossible to get staff sufficient to man some of the wards, that they might open it and thus relieve the overcrowding at Bellevue and what was then the old Kings County Psychiatric Hospital. The latter was a little rat-infested wooden building, where, if you were a visitor, you were obliged to go directly on the disturbed ward as there was no reception room. In this disturbed ward, Ward 21, I remember, the visitors and patients sat huddled on long benches, crowded in so tight that they had to sit at the edge of these benches in order to engage in private conversation with close relatives and friends.

The Manhattan State Hospital, which is on an island in New York City, is an eighty-year-old institution where sixty per cent of the patients were over sixty years of age. They were crowded into a slum which was just about as

THE ETHICAL STAKE IN MENTAL HOSPITALS

bad as any New York has ever seen — and New York calls itself the medical center of the world.

These are the things that go on in the centers of our civilization — the very core of American culture.

I don't know what the score is in Boston, except that three or four weeks ago, I heard Dr. Walter Barton, superintendent of the Boston State Hospital here, say over the radio that "it's terrible, it's pitiful, to walk through the wards and see patients so hungry and undernourished that they wolf down whatever food is placed before them."

He was talking about the undernutrition in institutions. And, on the same program, Dr. Kenneth Appel of Pennsylvania University, Professor of Psychiatry, called the state hospitals, in short, "monstrous and horrible places to be in."

How civilized are we? How different, essentially, are we who live in these centers of so-called civilization, from the people of the village of Belsen who said, "We are not to blame; we did not know about it; we did not do it."

But we do know about these things. We haven't even got the excuse of the witch-hunters of the seventeenth century — Increase and Cotton Mather — who were traveling up and down New England, preaching the witchcraft mania, finding witches all over the place, and paving the way for the death of twenty innocent people in the town of Salem. If you read the witchcraft trials of that time, you will find that, almost without exception, either accusers or accused or both were mentally sick people, suffering from hallucinations whipped up by the clergy.

But Increase and Cotton Mather had on their side, if they wanted to use it, the plea of ignorance as to this thing called witchcraft. And so, when they sent to their death innocent people in Massachusetts, they were doing it out of ignorance.

We are not acting out of ignorance; we know that

these people are sick people and that they are not being punished for sin or being possessed by demons, as our seventeenth century ancestors thought.

What are we doing about it? We are not killing them deliberately — no. We are not sending them to the gallows, but sending them to the grave and this is in the twentieth century American civilization.

A little more than a hundred years ago in East Cambridge, a forty-year-old school teacher, whose name is well known — Dorothea Dix — went down to the East Cambridge jail to substitute as a Sunday school teacher for a theological student who had fallen sick that Sunday. She saw there several patients who were mentally sick treated like criminals — placed in unheated cells in the dead of winter and shivering of the cold. She asked the cell-keeper, "Why do these people, sick people, stay here in unheated cells?" The cell-keeper said, "They're crazy, and crazy people don't need heat."

She insisted that these cells be heated, and the cell-keeper insisted that they wouldn't be. She took it to the East Cambridge court and got heat put in those cells. When she had found this at the East Cambridge jail, she went through the length and breadth of the state of Massachusetts to find out if other jails and other poorhouses were like the East Cambridge jail and she found that they were. You remember her pleading for decent, civilized treatment for mental patients which resulted in the expansion of Worcester State Hospital.

For forty years thereafter, this wonderful crusader went through the country, looking into conditions in our poorhouses and prisons and pleading for the placement of mental patients in hospitals.

If you read the psychiatric literature of the time, you will find that the word "hospital" had a kind of magic contagion. At that time, most of the mentally sick, as you know, were in the jails, poorhouses, and the prisons of the land instead of in hospitals, and the progressive people of the time thought, "If we could only get them into a hospital!" At that time, the word "hospital" became such a magic formula that the superintendents began to claim 80 per cent recoveries, 90 per cent recoveries, and 100 per cent recoveries of mental patients in their institutions.

But the point was that, a hundred years ago, this crusader did go through the length and breadth of the land, did get something like thirty new hospitals built as a direct result of her individual effort. When she died in 1881, the hospitals deteriorated practically to the conditions that she had seen in poorhouses and prisons forty years before.

As one who has followed humbly in her footsteps, I can point to places in this land, and document what I say, where conditions are just as bad as Dorothea Dix found in the poorhouses and prisons of 1841, '42, and '43. I say to you it does not become a society that calls itself civilized to tolerate that kind of condition.

And I say this, too, that, in many of the institutions I have been to, I have seen good, decent chaplains, trying hard to improve conditions as best they could; but I say frankly that I have also seen old "wheel-horses" of chaplains who do know what the score is in institutions they serve, never saying a word about it, never trying to make a contact with the community, tolerating these conditions which should not be tolerated this side of Hades.

I wonder what kind of spirit, what kind of religion motivates the chaplains of institutions who remain silent in the face of such social and ethical crimes as are committed daily in our mental hospitals.

I am of the profession of reporters — our job is to report; we haven't got the ethical responsibility that is vested in the clergy. Why haven't we got groups of clergymen — in every metropolitan center, at least — who will go into these institutions and who will give help to these superintendents and doctors who are struggling valiantly, many of them, with the meager appropriations they get from indifferent legislatures unsupported by any kind of public activities? Why haven't we got groups of clergymen in this city, in this community, in this country to go into these institutions to find out what's going on, to tell the public, to stand up as the champions of civilized care: "What you do unto the least of these you do unto Me."

I have seen many clergymen in many towns who haven't taken the trouble to visit institutions for the mentally sick within the confines of their own town. I say that of all of the occupations that are disgraced by uncivilized conditions in many of the institutions, I can think of none that bears the disgrace more heavily than does the clergy, because the job is a job of ethics, and that job must be done by the clergyman primarily.

And I say that the challenge of Dr. Brandt, who boasted proudly of killing 275,000 "lunatics and other useless eaters," is a challenge to our society. Let us put up or shut up. We cannot condone the shame by saying that we don't kill our sick people with weapons — neglect can be a social crime, too.

PART THREE

THE INDIVIDUAL AND HIS ENVIRONMENT

Psychological Problems in Childhood;
Adolescence, and Marriage;
The Problem of Grief

CHAPTER SIX

THE EMOTIONAL NEEDS OF THE CHILD

George Gardner

IN ACCORDANCE WITH THE TITLE of this paper assumed by me, I intend to confine my remarks to an outline of a point of view and an orientation in regard to the recurrent problems in the mental health of normal children.

In the first place I must emphasize that mental health is not a static condition which one attains at some particular time in life through the trials and vicissitudes of development through which one passes, and that once attained is maintained; but mental health is a dynamic, continuing growth process; and although we state in our slogans that mental health is procurable, it is not procurable as an entity fixed in time, but it is a day by day purchase which all of us must make.

I am impressed with the fact that mental health is a continuous process perforce of the manner in which we must view the human organism if we are to understand human behavior at all. I refer here to the biological point of view. Such a point of view emphasizes the fact that man is a continually reacting, continually responding individual, responding on the one hand to his inborn, instinctive drives for the fulfillment of certain needs, and responding to the factors in his external environment that aid or hinder in the fulfillment of these needs. I would stress here and now the phrase "aids of society" in fulfillment of these needs, because it seems to me that psychiatrists and educators are prone to emphasize and re-emphasize the prohibitions, inhibitions and demands of society as they affect the individual, at the same time giving little or no emphasis to the great resources existent in society for the actual expression of our instinctual drives.

Man, then, is to be looked upon as a biological entity, and as such he sets the task of his own development. The task, it seems to me, can be summarized in a general way by saying that the individual of necessity must work out the best possible bargain that he can between himself as a biological unit and himself as a social unit. This is not something accomplished at the age of three or five and then forgotten. Nor is it sporadically accomplished at adolescence or in the late teens and never again presents itself as a task or problem to be solved till mid-life or thereafter. The task of maintaining mental health (in its broadest terms) is always with us, and failure at any stage can make for unhappiness, inefficiency or even ill health in the normal individual at that moment, or lay the foundations for future disabilities based upon these unfortunate responses of the moment. With this general thesis in mind, let us turn, then, to some of these biological needs, the fulfillment of which constitutes the tasks of development of the child. In this way we can outline some of the orderly steps that are necessary in the maintenance of mental health. For if these needs are met in infancy, in childhood, in adolescence and adult life, the child is seen to develop normally, and a maturity is attained that is commensurate with the maturity demanded at each stage in the individual's development, and the adult stage eventually reached is a normal and stable one. If these needs are not met — that is, if the task set for the individual is not carried out — the development is seen to be jagged, with unwanted and harmful retardations and accelerations at certain points or in certain areas of his existence, or there may be a general and blatant immaturity in the total personality.

We may turn, therefore, to the emotional development

of the child for our cues as to the needs and tasks imposed on human beings if they are to remain healthy. We turn to the child not because his problems differ in kind and intensity from those of the adult, but because they are less complex in structure and not so far removed from the ultimate biological and physiological bases of all human behavior that we are unable to see their most vivid and compelling nature.

There are, it seems to me, three definite tasks in the attainment and maintenance of mental health in childhood, and these tasks tend to arrange themselves around three periods of childhood, namely, the pre-school years, the intermediate years between five or six and eleven or twelve, and, lastly, about the years of adolescence from twelve through the teens. We will consider these needs of the child and the nature of the milieu that can aid or deflect him in the attainment of health.

The first need of the normal and healthy infant as an insurance of his normality and health is the establishment of a firm feeling of security and love in relation to his parents. By security we mean the feeling that he is wanted and loved, and in turn that the physical needs of the hour and of the future will be met by these seemingly omnipotent factors that move in his vicinity. The child-parent relationship may not be aptly described as a parasitic relationship on the part of the child, with the child the parasite and the mother the host, but it is certainly a relationship that approximates it. The one aspect in which the parasitic relationship is not in existence is involved in the carrying out of the very tasks that we are talking about. In other words, the infant (and the young child) can and does do something about this host, and as soon as he reacts at all, he reacts with a view to establishing this all-important security of which we are speaking. What I am emphasizing here is that the child is not merely a passive, oral, receptive individual, though he may seem to approximate this condition in his early months of life, but he himself responds to positive and negative elements, and more particularly, as far as is our concern of the moment, he builds up definite defenses against the negative aspects of his environment.

What then are some of the factors, the more important factors, that aid or hinder the infant and young child's establishment of a feeling of security within himself as he lives within the home? We can list some of the more important of them. I have already spoken of the tremendous value of the actual and repeated demonstration of love for the child by the mother and father. It is not so many years ago, and still continuing unfortunately to the present time, that we in medicine, particularly in pediatrics, emphasized the tremendous importance of habit training and of the routine handling of the child. We placed the child on a time schedule in relation to his food and drink and the expression of his bodily needs and wants; but in so doing I am afraid we placed the child on a rigid schedule also as far as the important diet of love — mother love and attention — is concerned. I think we are gradually coming to see that the child is more important than the schedule, and also that to deny the free, spontaneous, and frequent expression and reception of love and bodily contact on the part of the mother and child is definitely deleterious to the mental health and emotional adjustment of both of them. We have been in the past too afraid of the mother's love of the child, assuming that an overemphasis of his needs would make for a fixation of the child's responses to a level of a passively recipient individual who never would exert himself or give of himself to the end that he might attain these interpersonal grants. Because of this, we urged the development of a parental attitude (or at least we complimented a parental attitude) that nearly bordered on the aggressive or obsessive type of parent. Such aggression or obsessive concern for minutiae of scheduling and control of mother love can be very easily interpreted by the child as a rejection, and certainly the latter is much more fraught with possible harmful effects than is the over-emphasis of the mother's love or of the frequent expression of the mother's actual enjoyment of her infant.

At any rate — to return to our problem of infant security — the task is set for the child. The task is set for him as a biological organism to react in some way to the love or the lack of love demonstrated by his mother, and he does this day after day, hour after hour; and the basic security or lack of it that he will show as an adult will be patternized in these very early years, and he will continually attempt to maintain or to change or to revise those patterns as revision is needed throughout his later development.

You will note that I have said little or nothing about the father as a factor in the establishment of the child's sense of security, and though his presence and his love may seem to be of little consequence in these very early years, they certainly are of great consequence before the age of nursery school or kindergarten attendance is reached. In the early stages the father together with the mother must set the tone of stability and security to which the child will respond. The very presence of the mother and father, the fact that they do not leave for any length of time, the expression of love of one for the other, and, finally, the lack of aggression of one towards the other are situations to which the child will make a standardized response, standardized as far as his future relationships with people of both sexes are concerned. Again, the love of the mother for the father or vice versa usually is not reflected in less love for the child, and this the child notes.

When we pass from the relationship between child and mother-father to the growth-provoking or growth-retarding situations that can be invoked in the family unit, we are immediately concerned with the three-cornered or four-cornered or even more-cornered relationship between the parents and any individual child, and all the other children in the family unit. These, in turn, extend the feelings of security or the loss of feelings of security beyond the simple relationship of mother and child. For example, equal love for brothers and sisters from the parents is an almost inherent demand of the individual child, though its opposites — jealousy and rivalry — may seem to be paramount as a response. However, the child is not secure when his jealousy and rivalry are rewarded by parental attention at the expense of his siblings, even though he may realize and relish the temporary triumph that such affords. Yet, on the contrary, he becomes more uncertain of their love, and more rivalry is engendered because he feels the probably transitory nature of his success at aggression. Only equal love for brothers and sisters will take away this uncertainty.

When one passes to the treatment of different children in individual instances, the child demands fair but not necessarily equal treatment of the children in the family — and there is a great difference between fair and equal. For example, no child is going to be secure unless there is an inequality of treatment of him in relation to his brothers and sisters, as such inequality is demanded by their differences in age. There are privileges of age even at two, three and four years, and such privileges must be respected by the parent if the child is to consider the treatment fair. There are other differences in day by day existence that require a fairness rather than equality of treatment as, for example, in the presence of temporary illness or disability, the fair response on the part of the parent may not be one which can be generalized throughout the sibling group at that time, and hence "fairness" must always take precedence over "equality."

Again, fair and consistent punishment in the form of loss of privileges to all children in the family is demanded in the interests of the child's security. Each of these words "fair" and "consistent" should get their due emphasis because there is nothing that can be so unsettling to the child as a deviation from either attribute and so lead to confusion and insecurity. I think I have never given a talk to parents or teachers or both without the question concerning punishment being raised. I have emphasized the loss of privileges as a method of punishment most effective, and with it I would emphasize again the necessity of the maintenance of an attitude of still loving the child when demonstrating a dislike of the child's actions that call for the loss of privileges. And, although at the present time no one advocates corporal punishment as the best method of inculcating good habits, I think it is necessary to emphasize that in the interests of the child's own inner feeling of security, it is necessary that he be punished in the way indicated above for errors in conduct. Otherwise, in the absence of any "punishment" whatsoever, two unfortunate things occur. In the first place, the child gets an entirely unrealistic view of life as it is to be lived day by day and in the future; but more important, it seems to me, he builds up an internal feeling of guilt which is not dissolved if the loss of privileges does not supervene. This is a very subtle mechanism, and the effects of these growing feelings of guilt are sometimes demonstrated only years later in the form of unexplained actions which seem to have the sole purpose of inviting the then felt need (or long felt need) for punishment of early deviations in behavior. I am sure that any psychiatrist will be taken to task in some quarters if he advocates that the child's omnipotence must be thwarted, but I feel that it is necessary to thwart it for the very reason that one's opponents would say it should not be, and that is, in the interests of the child's inner peace, his security, and his mental health.

If we now pass from a consideration of the direct parent-child and parent-sibling relationships to the attitudes regarding the more material aspects of his environment, it would seem that it is easily shown that the child demands a respect for his possessions — the possession of his own toys, own playthings, knife, fork, spoon, cup, clothes, etc. The modification that is necessary for growth as regards behavior in this area is, of course, the continual emphasis on the desirability of sharing possessions with siblings and others, but at the same time the actual ownership must be respected. The child's responses here again will be such as to determine in large part his later attitude towards the material things in his environment, his strivings to attain them, the methods of his strivings, and the use or lack of use to which he will put them once they have been attained. He works to establish these attitudes, and he will continually work throughout the rest of his life to maintain them if they are adjustive and healthy or to modify them if they are maladjusting and conducive to his ill health or unhappiness.

Finally, as regards the very young child, there are the fears and insecurity related to the learning process itself which have to be considered by all of us. It soon becomes evident to every parent that there is a definite, though sometimes subtle, conflict between the desire on the parents' part to provide learning and learning situations and the desire on the part of the parents to provide a protected environment for the child. In other words, it seems that almost everything in the child's environment about which he may be and should be curious can constitute a hazard to his physical well-being, and the ever present task of the parent in driving an even course between the two extremes of indifference or over-protection is a very difficult one. On the one hand, the child may be prevented from giving the responses necessary for his education and development in any realm, whether it is physical, intellectual or emotional, and thus there will result an inhibited, insecure child. On the other hand, the child may have all the freedom necessary to express his curiosity, to express his feelings, or to experiment in his environment, and by so doing may harm himself in such a way that learning again is hampered and delayed. In either case, definite blocks can be set which will become evident in his later school career and in his social responses. Perhaps it is in such situations that Gilbert and Sullivan's "little liberals," to whom experimentation and growth are the elixir of life, and "little conservatives," to whom both are anathema, are made.

In summary, then, this is the first task of childhood, to establish in the midst of all of these externals an internal feeling of security — a security that allows a continuing positive response to the people of his later environments. If the child does feel insecure, certain defenses, compensatory responses and over-reactions are established by him to take care of his needs in childhood. These defenses are useful at the moment; they are his only protection, and they may continue to be useful and workable for many months or even years. However, their application to analogous situations in later life, that is, situations entailing the response to individuals, may fail to be workable and may result in unhappiness and inefficiency. At any rate, it is safe to assume that a sense of insecurity established in childhood sets an additional task for the child and adult in later years. It sets limits to his growth and retards the attainment of that growth within those limits.

The second task of child development, and in turn a continuing, ever-present task in the maintenance of child and adult mental health, is the primary establishment of an inner control of aggression.

I need not emphasize that the human organism is endowed by nature with the drive to be aggressive towards its environment. In present-day thinking as regards this instinct, there is a tendency to divide aggression into two types, primary and secondary. The primary aggression is principally allied to the task of food getting and all of the self-preservative maneuvers that the organism can make in warding off danger, in incorporating elements needed for life itself, plus the elimination of noxious or harmful substances. Secondary aggression, that type of aggression with which, perhaps, we are more familiar, is that normal response to frustration that we observe in all individuals. It is impossible, of course, to develop in the family structure of present-day society without being frustrated time and time again. In fact, such frustration may indeed be a necessary factor for each step in our growth from infancy upward.

The first controlling mechanism in respect to aggression is the external control exercised by parents and others about us. The control is acquiesced in by the young child because of his fear of loss of parental love. In short, his first "conscience" is the *person* who stands beyond him in the figure of the mother and father. However, the individual child is endowed with the potentiality of incorporating, as it were, this external conscience, taking it up unto himself in the form of an internalized inhibiting mechanism that at first is a highly personalized set of inhibitions. In other words, he says to himself, "Mother says you shall not hit brother," or "Mother says you shall not get dirty," or "Father says you shall not leave the yard." Coupled with this internalization of the prohibition there is a concomitant development on the feeling side in that feelings of guilt are engendered which are aroused whenever this conscience is not obeyed. It is as if this incorporated person were able to be aggressive towards the child himself, and he fears this aggressive thing which is now recognized by him to be a part of his own make-up, and the power and might of *self*-punishment is established within him (for good or ill). However, you thus see that at first it is really the mother who punishes or the father who punishes even when it is the child who "punishes" himself, i.e., even when the child at first frustrates his own desires and controls his own aggression. These father figures and mother figures we carry with us throughout life, and they are continually exerting their influence upon our behavior.

However, because of this type of development, the task of continuing development now set for us in respect to our mental health is that task in development whereby we must gradually impersonalize our aggressive and destructive tendencies towards people around and beyond us who may frustrate or block us in the fulfillment of our wishes; but also we must, in the interests of our own mental health and happiness, impersonalize, or depersonalize, the controlling or thwarting mechanisms within us that might tend to punish us if we *did not* do so.

Let us take the first part of this task for our consideration of the moment, that is, the continuing need in all of us to impersonalize our aggressive tendencies towards external frustrating agencies. The child early demonstrates his aggression towards persons; he directs his hostile feelings and actions towards his parents, towards parent substitutes in the form of other relatives, towards older sibling, teachers, scout leaders, policemen or any other person to whose lot it falls to see that the customs and mores of the group are followed by him. His hate and his desire to inflict pain are in the first instances directed towards these as people. Gradually, however, in the middle years, that is, from six to twelve, this personalized aggression becomes directed against a more generalized set of people, such as against opponents in games, where the game becomes a stimulus for aggressive behavior, and primarily, of course, at first towards the person who is the "opponent." But by the very fact that he can hold the concept of a frustrating person as being an "opponent in a game," he has made a first dilution of his hatred through impersonalization. He learns that his aggression can be expressed against "generalized persons" only in accordance with certain protective and protecting rules and regulations. And in this connection, I am sure it is not difficult for you to visualize how, from time to time, the "game" or the "society of the game" breaks down or is disorganized by the very fact that the boy, under pressure of thwarting or being out-pointed, again returns to an infantile type of expression of aggression (which is directed towards a single person involved), rather than maintaining the more mature stage of development of which we are speaking, where he is aggressive (in sportsmanlike fashion) only towards the game requirements themselves. You see here the paradigm and model for the impersonalization of aggression or prejudice that must be accomplished by all of us if we are to maintain our mental health and, indeed, become socially healthy individuals. You see also in this simple illustration of the playing field how we can revert and "repersonalize" our aggressions in the manner that we used normally as infants.

You can see also, I think, that society provides, even for the young boy, certain restricted and controlled milieus for the expression of aggression, where aggression is held to be satisfactory by society as well as satisfying to the boy. Society also provides such satisfactory settings for the expression of aggression to us as adults, and in all of our discussions I think it must be apparent to you that the mental hygienist is convinced that the aim of our development need not be that we stamp out these instinctual drives in the interests of mental health, but rather that we control them and divert them and get for ourselves as biological organisms the best bargain we can with society in respect to their fruitful and constructive expression.

But there are other devices that the child uses in this task of gradually impersonalizing his aggression, all of which are used in some part by us as the task is continued into adulthood. For example, the boy is aggressive towards evil fantasy-opponents in the form of "bad men" personified by some far away race or hostile group, the evils of which he has become acquainted with by virtue of the conversations of adults about him. Certain fantasied groups (and I might add that to him they are not much more than fantasy groups, even though they have the name of the inhabitants of a definite country) do enable him to direct his aggression somewhat away from the persons in his immediate environment to the evils which these unknowns are supposed to perpetrate. Thus, his aggression is more or less intellectualized in fantasy, and becomes once-removed from parents, from siblings, and from those near at hand. But our aggressions must be even further impersonalized, and so it is that later they are inveighed against the evils in society itself, the social and economic evils and wrongs that we all try as citizens to rectify. Again impersonalized aggression is expressed in our work or in tasks and hobbies, probably sought unconsciously for the very purpose of allowing an acceptable expression of our hostility. And, finally, at the very pinnacle of our maturity and mentally healthful states, we fight aggressively against wrong principles of action and fight aggressively for all correct, humane, and Christian principles.

We should emphasize again that this task is not only the task of childhood. It is the task of all of us in our search for mental health, and we have outlined the various stages in progression from childhood up, in order that you may see both the potentialities for growth and progression and also envision the possibilities for periodic regression, when we are tempted to revert to infantile, immature, and unhealthy expressions of aggressions in their various personalized forms.

Now paralleling this needed and constant task of the impersonalizing of the external objects of our aggression, there is also the needed and constant task of impersonalizing the inner mechanism of control and self-chastisement which we have taken unto ourselves in this process of development. In other words, the inner feelings of guilt and aggression directed against ourselves that we sense in early childhood are, as I pointed out above, in the first instances and for a long time in childhood associated directly with a person. It is as if our first voice of conscience said, "It is *she* who will be aggressive towards me, and I feel that she will punish me." This inner fear of punishment we call our guilt feelings. There arises also with this guilt feeling a seeming need for punishment. Gradually, however, the inner conscience is no longer a group of individuals exerting their several influences, but it, too, becomes impersonalized in a succession of stages, to become at last a closely knit set of principles of right and wrong and values of good and evil which seem far removed from any particular, individualized person, but which none the less enable us both to act justly and to thwart our own desires without referring such frustration to any single person, external or internal. Finally, then, we have the individual who is an ethical person, who divorces his action from the imaginary presence of some person or some group of people, and his guilt arises purely from a sense of having failed to act in accordance with these principles, not because he failed to act in accordance with the wishes of some individual. The maintenance of this type of self-direction is again the hallmark of the mature and healthy mind, but again the evidences in symptoms that we note in our disturbed and maladjusted patients convince us, the psychiatrists, that we daily fight this struggle against the tendencies of "over" self-depreciation or too severe self-punishment at the hands of a too severe — too rigid — and occasionally too "personalized" a conscience. It is easy (as we say) to "regress" to infantile habits of self-punishment.

Finally, there are two more tasks of mental health which have to be dealt with by all of us and which developmentally reach their initial stage of intensity during the years of adolescence, and at that time, in turn, lay the basis for future problems to be solved or for future adult mental health. I refer here to (1) the problems involved in the control and sublimation of the sex instinct and (2) the problems involved in the final establishment of an actual independent adult status, the latter in turn being accompanied by an internal feeling of emancipation and self-sufficiency. As in the case of the other two tasks in mental hygiene, let us consider these at the chronological age when they are most in evidence, namely, in adolescence, and we will begin with the problem of the expression of the sex instinct.

It is a mistake that many of us make to assume that the problem of the expression of, or the control of the expression of the sexual instinct are thrust newly structured as problems at the time of puberty and only following the physiological maturating of the reproductive system. For in relation to the purely physiological and anatomical aspects of the sexual drive and the expression of the various bodily pleasures associated therewith, the individual in his earlier years has been forced by parental and social dicta to establish controls, and he has been limited to only partial expressions of these drives. These controls by parents and society have been directed at the many, varied, diffuse, infantile, and only partially developed components of the sexual drive in childhood, as distinguished from the complex sexual instinct as we recognize it later in its more localized, unified, and mature form. Adolescence, then, would seem to be merely a stage — though an extremely important one — in the direction of the instinct as it now has as its object the biological functions of reproduction. In short, adolescence seems to be the stage where the unification of all of the diffuse, pleasurable bodily expressions has to take place if the individual is thereafter to have a normal sexual adjustment. For example, some of the controls of the earlier independent segments of this complex drive may have been inadequate and have to be strengthened by inner inhibitions, or some of those types of child behavior that we assume to be more or less normal in earlier life will now take on the aspects of a typical or even perverse sexual behavior. Again, perhaps these controls which the child in his earlier years was able to establish were adequate for the time being, but are now seen to be inadequate when the strong heterosexual drive in adolescence supervenes.

Whatever may be the situation, we can be sure that in the interests of mental health and adjustment the adolescent has to establish or re-establish certain defenses against these inner drives. In most cases this is accomplished without much difficulty. On the other hand, due to the inadequate or too adequate (that is, too rigid) training of the child in early life, the adolescent may establish defenses against sexual expression that by their very extremeness and severity become quite disabling. These defenses of adolescence are commented upon extensively in the literature on child development. Examples of these extreme defenses are tendencies on the part of the adolescent to periods of shyness, sometimes in so extensive an area of his daily life as to make the parents and his family physician wonder if he is becoming mentally ill. Again, there may be an overreaction against these inner feelings in the sense that he becomes overconscientious, assumes that everything that has to do with the sexual drive or the opposite sex is bad, sinful, or evil. He may turn to endless intellectualizations of his problems, with an absorption in some new, radical or perhaps ultraconservative type of social order. He is absorbed in these new social orders that he constructs as the solution to alleged or actual economic and social problems, where in reality the conflict he is trying to settle is his own emotional conflict relative to the expression or nonexpression of certain individual needs and desires.

At any rate, whatever defense is established, it is extremely important on the part of the parents to recognize what the adolescent is trying to do by such maneuvers and thus, if necessary, to be able to help him, that is, to understand that these are the best possible defenses that he can erect at that time to control the increasing power and urgency of his instinctual drive. However, as in the case of all defenses, they themselves can become disabling; whether it is in the area of biology — for time and again certain species have overdeveloped themselves in certain defensive equipments and perished — or whether in the realm of politics, when nations feeling themselves threatened from within or without have erected defenses which, in turn, have led to their destruction. So, too, can we carry our internal controls and prohibitions to such a degree that the very thing we are trying to insure becomes destroyed in its own defenses.

A second point of importance in relation to these problems is that adolescence is not the only time when these problems will be presented for solution. It is merely that in adolescence the ever recurring problems relative to this instinctual drive are thrown into relief for initial, acute and critical solution; but you will note that thereafter not only the instinctual drive itself becomes a problem, but also the multivarious defenses which we erect to care for it may in themselves constitute problems that call for ever repeated modification in the light of our future development and growth throughout our adult years.

The second problem which is of great concern during the adolescent years, that is, the drive for emancipation and independence on the part of the individual, is also dependent upon and in large part influenced by the solutions that have previously been made in earlier life to the heretofore mentioned problems of security or insecurity, aggression or passivity. In other words, if the earlier adjustments in regard to these have been inadequate, the problem of adolescence and freedom from parental control, the overcoming of dependence, and the gaining of a state of self-sufficiency will be much the more difficult. Here again the internal pressures and the pressures from colleagues, from parents, and from society as a whole, insist that there be a solution to these problems in adolescence. It is as if a new drive had been implanted in respect to these problems, just as it is in the biological make-up of man.

Now the drive for adult status in adolescence immediately sets up certain serious conflicts that have been hinted at in various ways in our literature. On one side of the conflict there is a drive on the part of the child to be independent of his parents, to make his own decisions regarding his comings and goings, to choose his own friends, to determine his own academic and educational future. Everything about him insists that he shall assume these responsibilities, and he himself feels strongly that he should do so. On the other hand, there are always the fears that contemplated independence brings to his mind — the fear of losing the parents and all of the material and spiritual gifts that they can give him, the fear of the possibility of making wrong decisions, choosing the wrong type of friends, selecting the wrong vocation on the basis of some temporary whim. This conflict makes for the typical state of adolescence, which is best described as a state of continual indecision and fluctuation of needs and desires. It is, in short, the characteristic "obsessional indecision" of the adolescent. It is not necessary, I think, to point out again how important at this later time are the solutions to the problems of security that were made in earliest life. Nor, in turn, is it necessary to point out that educational, vocational, social or marital decisions and choices made now can be definitely *neurotic* choices, and that their influence on future mental health may be great. More important still, it is to be noted, is the fact that problems of dependence and independence, problems of aggression and passivity, problems of security and insecurity, are with us always.

I can best point out to you the continuing process relative to dependence and independence, love and security into adulthood by emphasizing briefly in this place the conflicting responses and reactions on the part of the parents (that is, adults) of the adolescent. They, in turn, wish for the independence and self-sufficiency of this child, but also fear the loss of love that a removal of his dependency upon them may create. They, of course, are subjected, too, to internal and external pressures in both directions, and here again their solutions to their own childhood and adolescent problems, and all that have followed thereafter, will in large part determine their attitude toward these children who are now attempting to become free from them.

Now in summary, you will note that I have outlined three main tasks of the developing organism that must be completed before the individual can take his place in the adult world as a reasonably mature man or woman of normal mental health. And though I have assigned the initial and the greatest concern for them in the main to the three decisive developmental stages in child development — the pre-school, the grammar school and the adolescent years — I would not have you feel that such problems are wholly concerned with any one era of development. They are present either in their entirety or in one of their component parts in all of the childhood years.

But of even greater importance to us, it seems to me, is the fact that these problems are not at all solved once and for all and set aside forever during our childhood. On the contrary (and here we must return to our original thesis) these are the ever present problems of mental health, problems that recur and are reactivated day by day — almost every day — and must be re-solved by us in the interest of our continued adjustment. These problems, of course, do not necessarily reappear in their original intensity, and surely they appear in settings where our increased information about this world can usually better enable us to handle them; but none the less they do repeatedly reaffirm their insistent needs and persistent demands, and thereby they demonstrate as nothing else can the uncompromising and unchanging biological bases of human action.

Our sense of security and feeling of being loved and wanted must not be lost to us in adulthood any more than they could be threatened in our infancy if we are to maintain our mental health and happiness. To what lengths we go to insure these feelings and to what extremes are we driven to avoid their loss! The burdensome defenses — even fantastic defenses — which we erect in our isolated personal relationships, in our group relationships, and as a nation in our international relationships — defenses to serve as bulwarks against feelings of insecurity — illustrate the power of the first solutions in our infancy, the power for good or for ill in our later years.

Closely allied to this problem of our security (so closely allied, in fact, that they usually cannot be separated as single problems) are the every-day problems of our aggressive instincts. Each day we express, control or resolve these feelings, each instance of which calls for new, however minute, techniques, subtleties, and differentiations as new situations are presented to us — but applied none the less to the never-changing instinctive core of matrix present in infancy. The exacting balance of external aggression (aggression expressed towards someone else) and internal feelings of guilt (aggression towards oneself) is demanded and met by us every day of our lives, and if the scales are tipped too much in either direction, we are miserable or we are delinquent or, as is usually the case, we are both. Here is the continuing struggle to impersonalize the aggressive acts of others, as they seem to concern us, and to depersonalize our own aggressive feelings before they are expressed — and, what is equally as important, while so doing to avoid that passivity, indifference, or even cynicism that is individually and socially so unproductive for either individual or social gains.

And, finally, there are the repetitious problems of our drive for independence and the maintenance of an adult status itself, both of which fight continuously with the infantile desire for a simpler and less demanding environment and the childlike yearning for a passively receptive and controlled state of dependence where all of our actions will be determined and all of our needs will be supplied by others — either by individuals, by relatives or by groups, or perhaps even by "the leader" or "the government."

Two things I hope, then, will be clear about the normal mental health of the individual, and they are both *points of view* regarding human behavior. The first is best called the "genetic point of view" whereby we mean that the present, current behavior of a man or woman (a cross sectional segment of it, if you will) can only be understood in the light of his past experience from infancy up — that is, it can be judged only in a longitudinal sense as it (the segment) takes its place in relation to those responses that have been expressed in earliest childhood. The second point of emphasis has been that mental health is a continuing process that has to be attained and maintained through an endless number of our responses day after day. We have, in short, to "work at" this problem of our mental health which in itself is a composite of hundreds of these momentarily adjusting or momentarily maladjusting bits of behavior, and victories gained today are but bridgeheads to victories to be gained tomorrow — and throughout our lives.

Discussion: MARTIN A. BEREZIN

What I should like to do is to reinforce some of the points Dr. Gardner has mentioned: I should like to point out certain clinical facts and examples, and, in the course of the discussion, to mention some repeated misconceptions which we must face constantly.

Dr. Gardner spoke of the "genetic viewpoint" — which means just a cross sectional understanding of the individual as he comes into our lives, for a person isn't just what he seems to be when he walks into a room. This cross sectional or horizontal segment, means that the individual is the sum total of his lifetime experiences. A little phrase I came across recently epitomizes in a very neat way this genetic viewpoint. That phrase is, "Past is prologue."

Dr. Gardner mentioned the phrase "day by day purchase of mental health." I think this is a very important viewpoint — namely, that mental health is not a static situation, nor is it a stagnant one, but goes on constantly; it is the ability to maintain a certain amount of emotional stability or mental health, and that that must exist constantly to form a dynamic process.

The word that we use for this day by day purchase, or hour by hour, or minute by minute purchase is homeostasis, and a kind of synonym for this is "equilibrium." What do we mean by homeostasis or equilibrium? Homeostasis is an attempt to maintain equal stability. The motivation of homeostasis is to avoid pain or ill health. We see this not only in emotional spheres, in psychiatric terminology, but it appears in physical conditions as well.

If I may, for a moment, try to present this viewpoint of homeostasis, I will take an example from our physical body which is constantly, moment by moment, maintaining the attempt to preserve equilibrium. An excellent example of this is the pH of the blood, referring to the acidity and alkalinity found in the blood stream. The chemical testing of the blood stream always finds it to have a pH value of 7.43. This is constant, but it is not a stagnant constant, it is not a static constant of 7.43; it is constantly changing. There are forces which attempt to make the blood more acid or alkaline. For example, certain foods we eat may have more acidity content when they get into the bloom stream. These will alter the pH value and make it more acid, but the blood won't permit this to go on this way. Therefore, certain solutions and

buffers in the blood stream immediately neutralize the
acid which has come into the blood and bring it back to
the constant pH value of 7.43. Likewise, the same thing
may happen if excess alkalinity gets into the blood — there
are buffers, substances in the blood stream, which will
neutralize the alkaline content, so that the pH value does
not change.

This is, in other words, a homeostatic principle in the
physical body, physical organism, and so, in neuropsychic
or mental health, there is a constant homeostatic strife.

Where there is any disturbance in psychic equilibrium,
this disturbance will manifest itself in symptoms referable
to the individual himself. Certain symptoms manifest
themselves in the peculiar, odd behavior of that individual, because you must regard the individual in three
spheres — thinking, feeling, and acting. The disturbance of
the equilibrium can manifest itself in any one or all three
of these spheres of thinking, feeling, and acting.

Dr. Gardner mentions that man's problems result from
two opposing forces: this is a conflict, and always means
two opposing forces. The two forces implied in Dr.
Gardner's discussion are the biological versus the social
strivings.

In this connection, I might point out that biological
values, biology, living organism, has existed, scientists tell
us, for about a thousand million years, whereas the social
strivings and the inhibitions and so on, or what we might
call the evolutionary development of man is only a few
thousand years old. So, we are still in the biogenetic stage,
still struggling to emerge from the dense biological and
archaic biological principles which originally motivated
living organisms. Attempt is being made by the development of the cerebral cortex, namely, reason.

This wide discrepancy in the age and historic background between biological and so-called social strivings

may make it clear that we can expect, then, not so much less emotional ill health, but perhaps we can understand more clearly that ill health does exist, and not consider it too remarkable as such.

Also from a genetic viewpoint one might observe the development of the individual in various channels of development. I would like to break this down, because we do see many individual differences. There are certain constitutional factors, and Dr. Gardner has mentioned the fact that there are physical and constitutional factors involved in the development of the individual. I would like to regard the development of the individual in four different categories or channels.

The first one is very simple, namely, the chronological development of the individual; each year, the individual adds another birthday to his life. Second is the physiological development of the individual; the physical or physiological is consistent with the chronological development, but here we already see, very often, individual differences. Some people grow, as it were, more rapidly than others in a physical sense. Sometimes we will see a child of six and will say, "My, he looks so old for his age." We might say the opposite, "He looks so young." We see it in adults, too. These are individual differences, but this is another kind of development that takes place in normal people.

Another and third area to watch, and observe, is the intellectual development. We are all aware that the child can't talk at birth, but gradually learns to talk and walk as part of the intellectual development, and that there are certain individual differences among people, intellectually, as well. The so-called "intelligence quotient" or I.Q. varies among people, again depending upon many other factors which enable the individual to develop intellectually.

Of course, the fourth is the emotional development,

and it is with this that we are mainly concerned in our discussion. Here we see also many variations and individual differences.

Finally, in all four areas, we arrive at a state of maturation, that is, adult life. Sometimes, in various of these stages, we don't achieve that adult status at all. We retain certain of our infantile strivings and problems, and sometimes we see so-called grownup adults acting like children. How often we have said that under certain circumstances.

A certain misconception in psychiatry which was mentioned by Dr. Gardner is the question of prohibition and inhibitions imposed upon the growing child. It has been so frequently asserted that the reason we have neurotic adults is because we have inhibited children; *ergo,* the implication is understood that if we remove the inhibitions, we will have a normal adult. Dr. Gardner specifically stresses the point that this is not so, and I should like to reinforce that point. It's a very bad kind of misconception.

A lot of people have tried, and we have seen some of the results of it, but I would like to assert here and now that I don't think that any reasonable psychiatrist ever said we should remove all inhibitions and punishment and so on.

Dr. Gardner said something about the rigid feeding schedule. I would like to say something about this, because the rigid feeding schedule can be an example of too strong an inhibition, which can be just as bad as no inhibition at all.

Interestingly enough, we know that if we permitted the child to feed as it wishes, we would see that the child develops a kind of rhythm of eating, a kind of rhythmic schedule of his own, which is an established schedule. In a program outlined for rigidly scheduled feedings, where the child is fed by the clock rather than by his

stomach, there is a certain rhythm which the doctor or
pediatrician or family suggests — feed the child every three
(2, 5, 8, or whatever it may be) hours first, then four hours
later. It's interesting to observe that this rhythm was first
taken from the child, who told us, "This is the rhythm by
which we eat."

This kind of reverse logic reminds me of something
I heard on the radio once about some Tschaikowsky melo-
dies. Many of you are familiar with the fact that a great
deal of popular music was written and taken from the
Tschaikowsky symphonies and made into beautiful songs,
and crooners sing them and swing bands play them and
so on. I think the climax came one day when I was listening to the radio, and an announcer said that now they
were going to play this melody, made into a special symphonic arrangement — a kind of going backward in taking
the symphony melody, originally arranged symphonically,
and putting it back into a symphonic arrangement. This is,
in a way, suggestive of what has occurred in the feeding
schedule for children.

Of course, we also have to realize that feeding an infant is more than just giving him food, for many things
occur at the time of the feeding of the infant. Most im-
portantly, with the feeding of food that he needs, goes
also certain handling and cuddling and affection which the
child likewise needs. It is interesting to know that some
experiments have been done along that line, to show that
the child needs the handling and cuddling and loving and
affection and warmth as much as he needs the food intake
itself. In feeding without the cuddling and handling, lo
and behold, a shock-like state set in, and the treatment
of the shock-like state was the cuddling and handling of
the child, who immediately then recovered. We also see
other psychosomatic disorders which so frequently occur
in children when they are not properly handled emotion-

ally. I know of a case of a little infant who, when being fed, was not cuddled and handled, but instead was held at arms' length by the nurse who was feeding the child, and the food thrown at him, as it were, the whole process taking about five minutes. Soon, the child developed crying and colic, and the more colic he got, the more he cried; the more he cried, the more colic he got. Finally, the nurse went to him, picked him up, cuddled him a little bit, and the crying and colic would cease, but at each feeding the same thing occurred. This went on for a week or two. Finally, we were able to get at the root of the difficulty, and the prescription consisted in having the mother hold the child while the child was being fed — not for five minutes, but at least a half hour or longer. In a day or two, the colic disappeared, but if this had been permitted to continue, one can see the beginning, if you will, of certain psychosomatic disorders which might have occurred later in the life of this individual.

It is also interesting to note that children who are uncertain of the parental love and affection will test for parental love and affection. They start with the unconscious fantasy or unconscious feeling that somehow, "Mommy doesn't love me. I'm going to find out." So they will wander into the living room, turn over an ash tray, and wait for the expected punishment. Perhaps this time Mommy doesn't punish the child. Surprised, he can't believe it, so he goes and turns over one of the flower pots and gets the earth all over the rug. Again, Mommy doesn't punish. Then, he goes and tips a table over. This time, she punishes him — it's a little too much for her. Then the baby fantasy says, "Aha — I knew it all the time. Mommy doesn't love me."

There are two factors involved in this kind of testing which we find very often. One is this need to prove that "Mommy loves me," and, at the same time, a kind of getting-back at Mommy, too, because the child knows Mommy doesn't like this. So, it serves the two purposes of testing and punishing Mommy for the way she treated him.

I mention this point because I think you can see that the next step may be the development of a delinquent kind of child. It also may indicate, too, a wish to be punished. I think most of you are familiar with the fact that many criminals actually try to get caught so they can be punished. Not only that, but some people who never even committed a crime will make confessions that they committed certain crimes. If you follow the newspapers whenever a sensational murder story develops, the police are usually at their wits' end trying to decide which confession is the real one because a lot of people have a feeling of guilt; they wish to be punished, and so they submit a confession as if they had actually committed the crime.

Dr. Gardner's point about fair and equal treatment is well taken. Sometimes, it isn't easy to decide how much loving a child should have and how much he shouldn't have; how much punishment he should have, and so on. Dr. Gardner mentioned the precarious balance in trying to maintain this relationship. So, it isn't so much the dosage that is given at a particular time that is important — it is the fairness and consistency of the treatment of the child by the parents, because the dosage, as it were, will depend upon many circumstances. It will depend upon the age of the individual, and upon the individual needs, and constitutional needs of the child as well. It is hard to lay down hard and fast rules.

Another thing that Dr. Gardner mentioned, which I think is also interesting, is the "father figure" which we carry through life. We see this in many subtle ways, many unsubtle ways, and many spectacular and dramatic ways, too. I am reminded of military service where we saw the men in the organizations, soldiers, who rebel against certain father figures. I cannot say they rebelled against the father figure merely because they rebel — I can speak only of those particular men who came to my attention and with whom I was able to work out this fact in all its clinical details. It is interesting to note that even the Army literature regards the company commander as a father figure, and the men of the unit traditionally, historically, write about "the old man" — a father figure, and the "old man" is told in turn that he must not refer to men of the unit as "boys" but refer to them as "men." In other words, "Don't be too strongly a papa to these boys in your unit." You see the implications of the symbolic equivalent of the father figure and children, and so on. The men in the unit are all brother figures.

Dr. Gardner also mentions the "dilution of aggression," the opportunity, in socially acceptable ways, of discharging aggression. An important and necessary social contribution in this discharge of aggression is the establishment of certain instances set aside for this purpose, for example, a playground. It is interesting that playgrounds have always been utilized for this purpose without the advice of a psychiatrist. People intuitively sense the need for this sort of thing. They serve a very important and useful purpose.

Again, in the question of discharging aggression, Dr. Gardner speaks of the internalizing or depersonalizing of the aggressive impulses. In speaking of it, Dr. Gardner mentions the "fantasy opponent in the form of bad men," and I should like to elaborate on this.

It is interesting that a very common example wherein the fantasy opponents are depersonalized, as it were, is seen in the avid reading of the so-called "funny" books that children read. I have heard it mentioned that there is another word in describing these so-called funny books or comic strips — in England, they call them "penny horribles," and I think that is a more appropriate name. In these penny horribles, the child finds Superman, Captain Midnight, and Captain Marvel, who are always the good people, and the villains who are very sharply depicted as villains. He knows who is good or who is bad, and the boy or girl who reads them identifies himself as the good and struggles with the bad and finally conquers. This is another important point that is always there — namely, the good fellow always wins. So that the child who is able to read these, identifies himself with the hero, works his way through all these aggressions, kills everybody he wants to kill off, and at the end he feels good — he is able to win.

I had a ten-year-old girl who recited a story about Snow White and the Seven Dwarfs. She continued to tell me the story as you all know it. She went on and talked quite easily about Snow White and the Seven Dwarfs until she came to the description of the witch, when she stopped. I asked why she stopped. She said, "I don't know, but I just thought of my mother."

Now, this is a kind of extreme example of the identification which some children may go through in the reading of these books. I know that there are many questions as to whether they should or should not read the books; there are a number of points pro and con.

Adults, too, will tend to achieve a certain amount of satisfaction by means of identification in working out certain aggressions and certain wishes of loving affection, and a certain satisfaction which we are able to arrive at in our society — for example, in our present movies in which, invariably, we have a happy ending, even as with the comic books wherein the boy has a happy ending.

Do we have evidence to show what can happen to the child who is brought up in a secure environment? We do have a lot of evidence, not only within our own society and our own culture, but we see evidence in other cultures, in other parts of the world where children are brought up characteristically with a certain amount of love and affection. It is significant to note, for example, that the natives on Okinawa, during the time of bombing, didn't get upset too much. They didn't have the reactions that our own soldiers had; they are a very secure people. We find in them a certain absence of psychosomatic disorders; we find an absence of crime. In a community of 50,000 or 500,000, in a period of 50 years, they had but one murder. In our own society, we have 7,000 murders every year and 14,000 suicides every year. We have a tremendous amount of psychosomatic disturbances in our society; they don't seem to have anywhere near the percentage that we have, although I don't want to be misquoted as saying that we should bring up our children and live in the same kind of culture that this primitive people do.

Finally, I should like to say a word about this question of normality or abnormality. Those of us who are actively working with people and their problems and children and their problems, reserve for the laboratory or study of the wards, mainly, all ruminations about normality and the theoretical conception of it. On the other hand, we must have a workable definition of normality or abnormality to use in our everyday work with children.

Now, I would say there are certain criteria of normality. The first one is an over-all one and has nothing to do with children as such, but all people. Behavior that is satisfactory to society and satisfying to the individual springs from a mentally healthy individual: this is just a general workable rule that I will use. If it's not satisfactory, it's not healthy, it's maladjusting — it is, if you want, disabling, or abnormal, if you wish to use that term. On the other hand, it may be acceptable and be resorted to day after day as a response and be satisfactory to society, but not satisfying to the individual carrying out that bit of behavior. Therefore, it may, in turn, be disabling to him as an individual, and, if you want, abnormal. That is one criterion for workable use.

To that, in relation to children, I would add the following criterion. Is the behavior of this child at this moment comparable to what you would get in 85 to 95 per cent of all other children at this particular stage of their development? In other words, in children, you not only have to re-create a great many of the reference relations to the disabling aspect in the individual child, but you must also have a great many references that have to do with that particular child development at various stages. So, if behavior does not meet that criterion, it becomes disabling, or, abnormal.

General Discussion

QUESTION: It is, I think, a prevalent notion in psychiatry now to consider normalcy what is average and, moreover, what is acceptable to society.

Dr. Gardner mentioned that the child may sublimate in a good way, which means acceptable to society. Now I think it is quite apt, in this place, to ask the question: is always what is acceptable to society good? Shouldn't there be some other criterion for goodness than just acceptance to society? Things that have been accepted in Germany during the Nazi period — they were quite normal for that time in that society. Are they normal? Are they to be considered normal, or should we consider society in a broader way?

What is good can be not normal; what is normal can sometimes be not good for certain places.

DR. GARDNER: You are quite right in saying that what is acceptable by a particular society may not be good, may not be normal. I would not confine a normalcy to one side of this dyad.

What I said is, "If it is simultaneously acceptable or satisfactory to society and satisfying to the individual."

As I say, I have to have a working rule to judge behavior as it comes to me in the clinic in this particular society and in this particular culture. Psychiatry will reserve a deeper discussion of what is normal and what is not normal for some place outside of the clinic room.

However, I think the men in the ministry and rabbinate and priesthood should know that we at least work with some sort of concept, though we are not very sure whether we are correct or not. I agree with you 100 per cent.

QUESTION: In a boy that has failed to grow and has remained small, what reaction would that tend to have upon his later life?

DR. GARDNER: There are two definite possibilities.

On the one hand, with some of these youngsters who fail to grow physically, they feel a strong sense of physical inferiority. There is a tendency, of course, for them to overreact against this, by being aggressive in ways that do not entail physical entanglement with anyone. They will talk a lot, be very boisterous, and unnecessarily aggressive in many ways.

A quite opposite and not unusual reaction is for them to become quite passive. They will take on this passivity as a method of defence against a seeming notion of inferiority. You cannot predict ahead of time, although you probably could predict if you had all the evidence in the background.

In general, I think the picture that one has of a physically inferior youngster is that he becomes quite aggressive, but he may not be aggressive in the obnoxious sense.

He may be aggressive toward his books, and become aggressive toward the knowledge that other people have and become an intellectually superior child. He can use that as a device against his feelings of inferiority or even insecurity. There is no way of predicting the way it will be, but what we have to do is get such a child compensation in socially acceptable ways.

QUESTION: We seem to know pretty well how to treat children and what is the proper way to bring up children. That is, books have been written about it, and we all seem to agree on the various proposals. What is wrong when we find the adult who does not treat the child properly?

Is it because parents have grown up improperly or are there other external factors that enter into it and make it almost too difficult for us to follow through on suggestions, recommendations, that psychiatrists give parents in the bringing up of children?

DR. GARDNER: I should say this: in the first place, I don't think parents do such a bad job in bringing up their children. On the whole, I think they do a marvelous job, when you come to think of all the possibilities for ill that there are in bringing up a child. I am not at all an alarmist in relation to parents. I think that parents are pushed around; pushed into the background; told to do this, that, and the other, that they are "doing this wrong," and "why don't they do this?" and so forth. I would say that, in most instances, parents do a good job, and I will add that I think parenthood is the most difficult job I know of. It is a twenty-four hour job that requires all of the resources that an individual can muster to take care of the day by day problems you mention.

I think the answer to the question you raise is inherent in the discussion that you give to the point; that is, that when parents fail they usually do so because they can't eliminate their own needs from the situation. I don't know that we could expect them to do that 100 per cent and do it 100 per cent of the time. They have not been analyzed; they don't know all their internal difficulties; they don't know what all these things mean to them. We do give them certain workable rules and regulations and then we know, or we should know, that they can only approximate those, and the psychiatrist himself, who is bringing up his own child, can only approximate. He tries to approximate them all of the time.

My feeling, in answer to your question, is that it is a continual process of education and re-education, one generation after the next. And who knows, to people a hundred years from now, these things we talk about may seem very archaic and part of an education of all of them from the earliest infancy up — so that they will be better prepared for the nuances in behavior which seem so disastrous in the child's development.

My feeling is that, unless the parents have some very grave, intrinsic, perhaps neurotic need that really requires psychiatric help, they do a fairly good job at this thing. It is only upon the extreme cases we see that we erect our theories.

I think if the parents fail it is generally because they get in their own way. Their own needs are being fulfilled by acting aggressively toward their child or by being overprotective of the child, or by their carrying out some disabling type of behavior in reference to the husband or wife in the child's life. It usually refers back to the earliest years.

QUESTION: When should parents seek psychological guidance for their youngsters? Does one have to wait until something abnormal or neurotic manifests itself in sharp contrast, or should that guidance be given from the start?

DR. GARDNER: When should children go to a psychiatrist or be taken? I would say, when they are disabled. I think the disablement criterion is the best one we have. The child with one nightmare, or nocturnal fright terror, is not disabled, but if it continues he is.

Disablement is not only on the repetitive side. Suppose it was of such a nature that it was getting in the way of his development at school? Suppose every day he was sick, every day he couldn't leave his mother to go to school? It is not only a symptom, and a pathological disablement, but it is getting in the way of his normal development day by day, so that those criteria could be applied.

QUESTION: Are most pediatricians aware of, and equipped to serve, the psychosomatic needs of the child?

DR. GARDNER: I think we are now bringing back to pediatric medicine those things which we find in child development that pediatricians should know about, and I think they are becoming more and more cognizant of the mention of these things. But it is a long, hard road that psychiatry has in relation to pediatrics or any other branch of medicine that is not psychiatry, because we deal with things that they are not accustomed to use. The tools we use are not syringes, not medicines, but verbalizations, feelings — they have to do with anxieties and intangibles — and it doesn't give the pediatrician a great sense of security or the feeling that he knows what's going on when you step out of the realm of preventive medicine, in relation to toxin and antitoxin, proper foods and diets, proper clothing, and get into such intangibles as emotional factors, anxieties and greeds, mothers' needs, childhood expressions and fantasies, and that sort of thing.

QUESTION: I think it is a common conception that great

works of art are the result of suppressed feelings of aggression, or of the suppressed sexual urge. If future generations become more and more "well balanced" and have fewer of those suppressions, what will become of great works of art as we know them?

DR. GARDNER: I don't think that art, music, and literature (and I think you probably have reference to music) will be endangered, for I think we will always have conflicts because our biological unit will demand expression that society will never be able to condone. At least it seems to me almost impossible to conceive of the biological unit getting full and complete expression of its needs and demands. Therefore, you will always have expression, if you wish to look upon art and music as that expression of energies that these men and women make into more symbolic creations.

The ideal of a conflictless society seems to me to be impossible from the biological point of view. I can't conceive of growth taking place at all without some sort of stimulation, some sort of frustration of the child and hampering of his inner biological drives. The child, or the organism, that is completely satisfied at every stage in its development would, it seems to me, be an abnormality in itself.

I don't think conflict will be eliminated to the extent that it eliminates creative art.

CHAPTER SEVEN

THE ADOLESCENT, HIS CONFLICTS AND POSSIBLE METHODS OF ADJUSTMENT

Lydia G. Dawes

IT IS WELL KNOWN THAT adolescent conflicts usually center around relationship with parents; love affairs; sexual impulses and how to manage them. Adolescence, one might say, is the halfway point between childhood and maturity. Psychoanalysis, as you already know, made the discovery that during the first five years of a child's life, basic patterns are laid down, characteristic responses and ways of reacting emerge which have far-reaching influence on the later character and mode of reacting that one sees in the adult. Just as earlier, the child's series of naughtiness and unpleasant habits were shown to be no chance happenings, so we know that what, at first glance, looks to be a hopeless jumble of contradictory emotions and attitudes in the adolescent, is actually the repeating of earlier patterns. With the maturation of the reproductive system, a regrouping and re-aligning of the instinctual forces also takes place. A silent inner battle begins in which the ego struggles anew for dominance over these fluctuating instinctual forces of which the most powerful is the genital instinct. In adolescence this instinct occupies the center of the stage, surges forward and forces the young person to recognize it and manage it. Old sexual wishes, repressed since early childhood, emerge, usually in the form of daydreams. Most of the difficulties which we observe during this phase of development are due to the fact that the young adult is attempting to gain control and manage this most powerful of all the instinctual urges. In this struggle he often feels completely alone and helpless. He also feels guilty and knows that he somehow must, at all costs, keep his secrets to himself to gain his independence. He senses also that he must detach himself from his earlier childhood dependence on his parents' strength and he must make his own decisions. Earlier parental attitudes have built a barrier which makes it impossible for him to talk freely at home about his feelings. So he begins to act in a bizarre way. Often he will form new attachments to people outside the family circle who, to the parents' consternation, seem to exert a very powerful influence over him. They stand helplessly by, unable to break the attachment. The parents have some cause for worry if the young person makes an attachment to an undesirable person at this time.

The average adolescent is preoccupied with the opposite sex, either openly or in fantasy. In the usual course of development one member of that now mysterious opposite sex seems to be the true embodiment of "everything that is excellent!" Again the parents are alarmed. They are realists and see clearly that the fantasy of the young person has clothed this object with attributes that are not present. The over-evaluation of the chosen object irritates them and they feel often that the boy or girl has picked the wrong type to love. The more they try to dislodge his interest, the harder and faster he holds on to his new choice.

The great upheaval going on within the adolescent, as one may well imagine, exerts in turn a powerful influence on, and provokes a variety of responses from, the parents. On their side, they, too, are going through a very difficult time, because the child they thought they knew so well has suddenly become a most difficult and unpleasant stranger. Gone is the obedient and lovable child of yesterday. In his place is a changeling, — an unruly, often cruel and sarcastic, over-critical person, who may be meticulously clean one day and dirty and disorderly the next. He seems to have lost all modesty and sympathy and to have become unfeeling and hateful. "Although too he is capable of great idealism and self sacrifice"[1] and can readily pivot from this behavior to attitudes indicating the egotistical self-interest which is usually uppermost. Whimseys and vagaries are legion. There is so much emotion generated on both sides that the very important problem which confronts the young individual is all but forgotten. One might say that it has been completely overlooked in many instances. But how can anyone think clearly during a bombardment? The adolescent is being shaken within by his urges. He is in conflict and feels guilty and miserable for the aggressive targeting of his parents, which in his heart he realizes is unjust. Yet he stubbornly continues to bother them and blame them for all his troubles and his misery. The parents, in turn, are hard put to it. They feel angry and hurt because all their efforts seem suddenly to have come to naught. Just when they expected to find a companion in the young boy or girl, they have, instead, a scowling, sour, over-critical, know-it-all young person who demands more and more clothes, more and more pocket money, is inconsiderate, who keeps late hours, keeps everyone waiting, who uses the phone or the car without consideration for anyone else, who turns on the parents, and seems, as one mother said, "to hate our guts."

We might pause a moment and ask, "Why does the adolescent use these methods to fight something which is normal and natural and happens in every individual?" We have to recall that, during childhood, he has been busy building and strengthening defenses against all the forbidden instinctual pleasures which suddenly threaten to overwhelm him. The methods used by the mother in curb-

---

[1] Freud, Anna, *The Ego and the Mechanism of Defence* (London, 1937), p. 149.

ing these instincts when they first appeared have already laid down definite patterns of response. Now, when the forbidden urges appear again, the young adult becomes able at last to express his negative feelings. These were repressed first during his training period when he was small and helpless. He apparently gave up habits during this time which met with his mother's disapproval either because the wish to keep her love or the fear of her disapproval or punishment made this expedient. When confronted again with the same sort of situations that plagued him earlier, he attempts to free himself once and for all from the highly charged emotionally toned past experiences. For years he has endeavored to comply with the demands made by his parents which concern his instinctual urges. Often he has been unable to do this completely. Now he is again in a difficult position. If he gives in to the urge, he suffers from a guilty conscience. If he attempts to repress the urge and avoid the torment of a guilty conscience, he is in danger of developing crippling hysterical, phobic, or compulsive symptoms. In either case this turmoil makes him difficult to live with. Therefore, all sorts of reactions can be observed if one looks closely at the average adolescent. Usually, the attention of the parents and educators is directed at the symptom in the spotlight, without taking into account the more powerful forces which are behind the scenes. So we find endless variations in the presenting patterns of this age; the shy and timid young people are inclined to daydream a great deal and often present an irritating slowness and lack of co-operation which drives the parents to frenzy. Others are more courageous and begin clumsy flirtations which may have serious consequences. Others proceed to overt sexual acts and make the first steps toward delinquency. The parents are usually unable to handle these problems objectively. No one can hurt or be so harshly cruel in seeing defects in adults as the adolescent. The parents are subject to miscroscopic examination by their offspring, which, in my experience is so searching that they are unable to stand it without a great deal of counter-affect being mobilized. It is small wonder that even a closely-knit relationship between parent and child, under the severe strain that happens during this period, begins to crack. Painful as it is for the parents, if they can detach themselves from the turmoil, they can recognize it for what it is, — a step forward toward maturity. The stronger the attachment was in the first years, the more difficult the child is at this time. He uses every weapon at his disposal to bring his parents into a bad light so that he can hate them. Never does the young person feel so alone as at this time — never so friendless nor so frightened. Sometimes the parental figures, more or less sure of themselves through all these years, become panic-stricken. They are afraid of this stranger. Small wonder that they, too, reach for ammunition which will protect them from showing the deep hurts that the children have given them. One woman put it, "I am so angry and so hurt that I come out of myself without knowing why, and behave in a most disgraceful manner." Another woman described beautifully what happens in hundreds of homes in the 'teen age. She began by saying that she was miserable and guilty and she was "failing her daughter." Her daughter was sixteen and very pretty. This young girl she no longer knew. Her lovable child had disappeared and in her place was an arrogant little hussy whom she felt was a powerful rival, competing for her husband. Daily she was put in the most unflattering light by the girl. No matter how hateful she had been five minutes before, when her father appeared she turned on the charm. The mother was unable to recover so quickly and her bad temper was in evidence. She began to hate the girl because her husband indulged the daughter in every way and always took her part, blaming his wife for lack of understanding. What changed this care-free little girl into a powerful rival for her father's love? What happened that he in turn seemed to be behaving like a man who has suddenly discovered a very charming girl? Is the mother right that there is just a shade of some-thing else appearing in the father-daughter relationship? Why does she show her very worst side? Is she right to worry? We would say that she is right — not because she is witnessing a passing phase of growth in which her daughter practices her new-found charm on a safe ad-mirer, but because of the mother's own response to this natural phenomenon. This mother was unable to step back and watch her daughter with tolerance and even amuse-ment, because she was actually afraid that she was losing the love of her husband. Her irritation with the girl be-gan to widen a breach which might have serious conse-quences for both, because if home becomes an unpleasant place during these years, the girl may turn to the streets for comfort. The same is true, of course, for the father's relationship with his son.

Let us look at a potentially dangerous situation of this sort: A short time ago I saw a young woman of high intel-lectual promise who had reached the age of seventeen. After years of studious application with a set of straight A's in college preparatory school and a very good start in one of the Eastern colleges, she suddenly came in to the dormitory one night at four A.M. A serious investigation took place and she was suspended. The parents came to me very distraught because their young daughter had been out with a young man until this hour of the morning. They were very puzzled why this supposedly well-integrated girl had done so bizarre and dangerous a thing. In a short time the whole story came out. The mother had been struggling for several years with a difficult adolescent girl who wanted her head but was unable to manage it, so to speak. She had stayed out several nights and there had been scenes at home, with promises "never to do it again," and the father had definitely taken the side of the daughter because he felt that mother was too strict with her and that if she was reined in too tightly, one day her instinctual forces would cause her to bolt and do something unpredictable. He was frank and open about his own early escapades, which were common knowledge to the girl. The mother, on her part, said that the girl would wall up and refuse to discuss anything with her. She told how many years she had worked to help this girl to get into college. Now her daughter had thrown it all over. She was so bitter, "I hate her," she said. "I can't bear to look at her. I just want her to stay away." Then she cried bitterly. This woman's response was not pathological, but it was unwise, because it further complicated the situation. It is natural, when one has put in a great deal of time and effort, as any mother does in rearing a child, that the time comes when she feels that she has done her work well and she can let the child go. Then when the child disappoints her, as this one did, she has a massive response of which she is very ashamed and guilty and which drives her away from the child at the very moment when that young person needs support, and love, and understanding. It was interesting that the mother had no memory of her own adolescent struggles. After seeing the girl, we (the parents and I) could again meet, and it was possible to bring the girl's problem into focus in an atmosphere where their intellects could function without the emotional bitterness and mutual recriminations that had been obscuring the issue whenever an attempt was made at home to talk things over. The mother's central fear had been that the girl had gotten into some kind of a sexual entanglement with the young man with whom she had been out until four A.M.

The father said, "Well, what if she has been? I expect she has to learn just as I did." The girl, on her side had this to say: "I met him, the night was beautiful and warm. I did not know him very well, but he was a very decent fellow. We decided to take a walk and see all the historic points about the city. It was much more fun than going on a sight-seeing bus, and we had a good long time to talk. We walked miles and forgot all about the time. I was more surprised than anyone when I got back to the dormitory and discovered that it was four in the morning." This may sound fantastic but the curious, dream-like quality of this experience was evident as the girl talked.

If we look into the girl's past we see that the mother has no cause for alarm as far as the sexual entanglement goes. The girl was still so naïve and unawakened that she was treading on air as she walked along with the young fellow. Instead of heavy necking and prompt return to the dormitory, which is much more frequent, this girl followed the pattern that had been laid down when she first met the strong instinctual force within herself. Her mother had said, "You must wait until you are grown up." That is what she was doing unwittingly, she was waiting. But there was a note of defiance also, because she felt again that strong instinctual force stirring within and so she took matters into her own hands. That is why the mother's aggressive response is understandable. The mother allowed the girl to come to me and the warm relationship that had originally been directed toward the mother was now very useful in our relationship because I could clear up the girl's tangled ideas on many topics (sex matters included) and help her over a difficult spot. She was reinstated at the college and she said, "Will you tell my mother that I am very sorry to have caused her so much pain. I was silly and I didn't think. Why does growing up have to be so hard? I am the sorriest for her.

I can still see her face, all drawn and tired. I really didn't mean to do it; I don't know why I did it, but you can tell her she does not need to worry about me. I won't do anything wrong." The last report was that these two were getting on quite well. The mother has allowed the girl to take over her own responsibilities. The reality shock that the young girl got when she found the sudden disapproval from an impersonal source seemed to give the last stimulant which was necessary for the girl to make the most important step forward, to realize that she alone, and no one else, is responsible for her conduct; that she must modify her behavior and take reality into consideration or take the consequences of her thoughtless actions.

Now let us look at another typical adolescent problem: Joel, a senior in high school, was sent to me because he was so very rude and overbearing at home that his mother and his young brothers suffered intensely. Also, he was failing in school. His father had died a year earlier and he had been very attached to him. This father had been a very busy, alert, but quick-tempered lawyer. The boy had been interested in law for years and determined to follow in his father's footsteps. The mother, on her own admission, had been extremely jealous of this boy because father had preferred his company to hers. After the father's death, the boy went through a depression. He was moody, he didn't care to go with his former companions, and his school work began to be poor. Any reminder from his mother that his father would be disappointed brought a snarling retort and impudent rejoinders. The mother told me that if she did not get some relief from this boy she would have to put him out of the house. He watched her comings and goings like a hawk, he cathechized her if she came in five minutes late, he accused her of neglecting the family when she went out in the evening, he made scenes at the table — complaining

about the food, and in every way making himself obnoxious. The worst scenes occurred when she asked him to
look out for the two younger brothers when she went out
in the evening. He was usually pacing the floor and when
she returned he made caustic comments, saying she was
no good. The mother said, "He is so changed that I can't
do a thing with him, and my life is one long misery."

The boy came to me over a period of months. He said
he hated women, they were no good. (He had been very
attached to his mother as a little boy, cried and clung to
her at kindergarten age.) He never could see why his
father married his mother anyway. If he didn't take over
at home, the house would go to pieces, his mother would
be out all the time, as a matter of fact. He lit a cigarette
with shaking fingers and let his youthful beard grow
enough so that he could make a scratching sound with
his thumbnail as he talked to me. He was full of great
plans for the future. He was a very big fellow. The day
he brought a pipe with him and choked trying to light it
followed a very bad scene with his mother the night before. When I said I always admired a man who smoked a
pipe, he suddenly broke down and cried. He said, "What
is the matter with me, Dr. Dawes? I'm terrible to my
mother. I don't know what makes me act like that." I
said that he couldn't seem to decide whether to be a baby
or a grown man. I told him his mother had called today
and said she would not pay any more because he was
worse than when he started. She said he would not get
up, would not pick up any clothes in his room, that he
was unbearable in the house, etc. He turned and said,
"Will you tell me something, am I crazy?" Then he told
me how he had been frightened by his own urges, how
he had knotted the sheets in his bed to keep from getting
too comfortable and thinking about girls, how frightened
he was of his thoughts and his feelings, how guilty he felt

when he did what he wasn't supposed to do, and so he even dragged up experiences (homosexual, sporadic — when his father died) and what he had done when he was a little boy. I asked what he was going to do about it all. He said, "I feel so much better now that that is off my chest and I'm not crazy, that I don't care if she doesn't pay. I'm going to get a job and come myself."

He did come. He got a job after school. His school work began to pick up, but he was afraid to show his new self to his mother for fear of ridicule. Some weeks later he did not come for his appointment, but his mother telephoned that there had been such a change in the boy that she thought it was a good idea for him to pay for his treatments. As a matter of fact, he had not paid for the last three. He had a better job, but he asked her to say he could not keep his appointments any more. I didn't hear from him again until the Saturday before Mother's Day when he appeared in my office without appointment. He was dressed in his best clothes, was freshly shaven and he handed me $3.00. He said, "I earned it myself, and I have just been to the University to register for next year. My marks are high enough so I will be able to get in. I wanted to get here so you could use this as a present for Mother's Day." I asked what he thought I should buy. He said, something for myself. I suggested a box of candy and he said, "Yes, and you should eat it all yourself and when you eat it, remember that I think of you as my real mother." He got fiery red and dropped his hat. Some months later the mother said that she was ever so grateful, that the boy had steadied down and she wondered if, after his father died, did I think that he might have tried to take his place. "You know, his father was very quick-tempered and he often used to bawl me out when I was out. Anyway, his school work is good and he cleans his room, and is no more trouble at home. Whatever it was, I'm glad it's over."

Some things that would be worthy of consideration at this point are the following: When the child is small, the parent can step in and stop any sort of behavior which seems to be injurious to the child or which is especially distressing to the parents. When that same child reaches puberty, the aggression which has been pushed out of sight through all the difficult first years has been lying more or less dormant and flares into the open, either in outspoken defiance, or passive resistance to the parental suggestions or orders. For example, if the young boy or young girl neglects his person or his room or clothing, he seems to say, "Once you could stop me from being dirty, but now I am big and I will be as dirty as I like and you cannot do anything about it." That is perfectly true. During this stage of development the child's own ego has to take hold of the responsibility of his own actions, and this struggle between the parent and the child which is very frequent gradually diminishes as the child steps further along the road to adulthood. Positions actually seem to be reversed at this stage, because the parents are the helpless ones and the child seems to be the one in control. However, these curious phenomena that are common to all adolescents probably are the outward evidence only of the great upheaval within, and it is as if the parent were used at this point as a target. The "you can't make me, and I'll do it myself" struggle is in direct proportion to the methods used by the parent in training the child through the successive stages, oral, anal and genital. The patterns of behavior that cause the most trouble at this stage are not there by chance, they are evidence that the struggle was never entirely mastered by the child in the early years. The length of the duration of this struggle is in direct proportion to the methods used in controlling the instinctual force when it appeared in the first place. The dovetailing of the parent-child relationship in those early years is still here, but in a disrupted form, and the parent often seems to spin with a whirling current of thought and feeling which surfaces abruptly in the adolescent. He automatically responds the same way he responded earlier (in similar situations, e.g. feeding, toilet training, masturbation problem) because these are actually brief reappearances of earlier conflicts between parent and child. The one great difference in adolescence now is that this time the parent has to step back from his controlling role and allow the young person to master instinctual desires and forces himself. Parents need not have so great a worry as they do about the whole topic of masturbation, because every young person wants to grow up and in an average case the young boy or girl gives up this activity because he, too, likes to grow up, and love for another individual helps him. Many of the gang activities are the manifestations of the individual's feeling that he needs support and a chance to compare himself with other people of his own age who are struggling through equally difficult times. Probably the new-found urges can better be fought if they gang up against the common enemy. Therefore, we find the ardent man and woman haters in the adolescent groups, of boys and girls.

The most difficult part is the parents' role in this stormy time. The more detached and adult the parent can be, the more objective sympathy and understanding he can offer the young person, and the less he descends to the level of the boy and girl and fights with him, the more gratifying it will be to him later to find that all the years of sacrifice and care and love that he has put into the rearing of the boy or girl will be repaid, by seeing that the young individual actually is able to free himself from his infantile attachments and enter into a richer, fuller and more mature relationship.

Parents who become bitter, who get angry when their boy or girl seeks out an older man or an older woman to whom they can talk and unburden their souls, should look a little closer. They will usually find that the person to whom that boy or girl has turned and begins to copy as a model is no one to be jealous about, but a reflected image of the child's inner model who has been there since early childhood and for whom the original sitter was the parent himself. It seems strange that the young person fights his inner fears in this way, but on closer examination one will see that it is actually so. It is a very painful time too for the young person. One young boy said, "What good am I now; I'm too old to sit on my mother's lap and I'm not old enough to take out a girl, and nobody wants me around." A young girl said, "Why does my mother yell at me? Doesn't she know that part of me is still a baby? I know I have breasts and my period, but I can't grow up all at once. Big as I am I would like to crawl on her lap; I feel so funny. And nobody understands me."

If there is too much parental interference in this stage, the inner conflicts are again suppressed and the young person does not make the important step forward but remains dependent and attached to the parents, develops neurotic fears or severe learning inhibitions, work inhibitions. The young people usually feel that the parents have changed, but as they grow up a little bit more they realize it is their own viewpoint which has changed, that these very human beings are full of faults, and if they were not, life modelled on infantile over-evaluation of parental figures, would be very difficult to live up to. As they understand themselves more they become less bitter and less intolerant of their parents.

In closing we should remember that in early life up to

adolescence the parent is actually in control and acts as a counterweight in helping the child manage his own instinctual forces, but during adolescence it is necessary that the parent give up this position and that the young person take over completely the control of his own instinctual life. The adolescent has to put his own house in order, so to speak. All the old conflicts which surge up from below have to be mastered. This is a big piece of psychic work and is energy-consuming and difficult. He also has bodily changes, which I have not mentioned and with which you are all familiar. Therefore, we must be patient with him and remember that usually, as the little four-year-old said, "he is able to manage." There is nothing static about the inner world and if the parent could stand back and watch the movement and change taking place before his eyes, and realize that it is a very necessary and important piece of growth, this painful process for both parents and child could be viewed in a more objective fashion. If the work has been done well originally by the parent so that he has given his boy or girl a set of standards of what is decent, he does not need to fear that while nature is busy changing the child's body into an adult's, that the governing part that he has so carefully built into the child will cease to function.

General Discussion

QUESTION: Can't we as parents, adjust our psychological attitudes, our homes and social connections so as not to cause these conflicts in our adolescent boys and girls?

DR. DAWES: In response to this question one might say that we can only approximate such an adjustment because we are dealing with many unknowns, and because we are all human. Probably every conscientious parent strives toward such an ideal picture of himself. If I gave the impression that the parents alone were at fault, I did not mean that, because the adolescents are difficult and I have great sympathy for the parents.

For instance — during the course of an analysis, when the parent is on the couch, one sees all the factors, both past and present, that contribute to his mode of behavior. Sometimes, for instance, his child unconsciously represents to him a rival of some sort. The jealousy then mobilized is not recognized by the parent. Instead, the child is criticized or scolded because of this unconscious feeling. In its place come frustration, hopelessness and disappointment in the child. The parents, unaware of what motivates their own behavior and driven by forces within themselves, are in a state of confusion.

If the relationship between child and parents gets too bad, I suppose the parents usually come to a psychiatrist for help. The parents are then aware that something is wrong. I think it is a healthy sign that they are.

Display of emotion is not to be condemned. However, misdirected emotions are very dangerous. I have seen some homes where every parental emotion is repressed. I don't think that is good, either. One child at the Judge Baker Clinic came from such a home and said, "I wish I lived in South Boston. I know somebody that throws plates when they feel like my mother and father do. Instead of that my mother and father just sit there and give me a fine lecture, and that makes me feel like a worm."

I am not sure that we can completely adjust our psychological attitudes. But we can learn to be critical of our attitudes and our own behavior, as well as the behavior of our children.

QUESTION: You mentioned difficulties of learning as one

of the results of adolescent turmoil. Would you care to say something more about this.

DR. DAWES: That is a very large subject and one of the problems that I have been interested in for a good many years.

It would seem to me that learning difficulties are aggravated in adolescence, but that they do not start in adolescence. They originate way back in the child's first years, when his curiosity, which is a very powerful stimulant for learning, is diverted from its original aim. This aim was the acquisition of knowledge concerning the origin of life and the difference between the sexes, the answer to such questions as, "Where do I come from?" "Where did you get the baby?" and so on.

If the parents, in attempting to answer the questions, have given the child the impression that one must not talk about such matters, then repressional curiosity occurs with a displacement of the conflict into the "learning field." This means that everything new to be learned is also taboo. In other words, the child tries to comply with the parents' demands, suppressing all curiosity.

I can give you an example. (I don't want anybody to think that I am criticizing any religion, because if I cannot speak freely I am in the position in which parents sometimes are.) I remember a little girl who came to my office. She was eight years old and very intelligent but she was also a day-dreamer. She could not read a simple page. So I sat down with her, and we began to look at the words that she couldn't read. She allowed me to have a pencil to take down the words, and I noticed that she made very many mistakes. As I showed her the mistakes, I said, "Why don't we go looking and see what this means — every time you come to 'cat' you read 'kitty.' " She said, "I know what that is." She went on to tell me about her cat at home. The year when this trouble started, she opened the clothes-press and found the cat with ten kittens. She tried to find out where the cat got the kittens and so forth, and she couldn't get anywhere. Mother said, "Don't talk about it — it isn't nice," and so on. I said to her, "Where did your mother get the new babies?" She said, "That's all right. They came out of her." "Where do you think the cat got the kittens?" She said, "Out of her, but how could she hold ten?" I said, "In a little while, we'll talk about that." Then she said, "You know, I am not supposed to talk about this because I tried to find out about this before, and Sister says that when I think these thoughts they are not good, and I should think about the shamrock." "About the shamrock? What's the shamrock?" She said, "Father, Son, and Holy Ghost." I said, "But why does she say that?" "I don't know." This child's preoccupation with forbidden topics passed for day-dreaming. She restricted herself, following her mother's prohibition, "You cannot learn anything new." Hence her inability to read.

I think this example is similar to difficulties in learning that we find later in college students. The child tries to do what the loved one wants. The child represses one thing and in its place comes an inhibition in the learning field. It is as if the parent still said, "You can talk about anything else, but not this." After a while the connection between the original forbidden curiosity and conscious interest in learning new facts is repressed, so that everything connected with curiosity is taboo.

It is surprising what an amount of knowledge seven and eight year old children have on all these topics, but they hide it in the same way that parents hide knowledge from the children. I very rarely meet a child who is not pretty well versed in most of these subects. When he is in an atmosphere where he can expand and talk freely, he does so.

Now then, in adolescence the great urge "to know" comes again. Adolescents are curious about the opposite sex and curious about their sexual instincts. They want to know all about intercourse and about all kinds of things, and they have a great deal of knowledge. But if the original repression has done its work well, a "learning inhibition" is the evidence of its existence.

QUESTION: Would you tell us a little about the antagonism between girls and boys in the early teens, and what it means?

DR. DAWES: As we observe it, they seem to be one way or the other — either all for or all against. I suppose that depends on the early training and the strength of the impulses in the child.

You notice it with boys — "Bosh! They don't want anything to do with girls." The girls gang up together in clubs, usually, or groups, and discuss their feelings about the boys and talk about all these mysterious things — each one gathers a little piece and brings it so that they get knowledge that way, you see. The boys are excluded because the talking together is exciting. Anna Freud says that with children, "talking is like doing." That's why I wondered about the advisability of giving lectures on such an explosive topic as sex to children in mixed groups for they are usually struggling to keep this excitement controlled. I think it would be better to give the information to them in separate groups — not to mix the two sexes.

CHAPTER EIGHT

THE PROBLEM OF GUILT IN THE ADOLESCENT

Paul Johnson

GUILT FEELINGS ARE MOST ACUTE in adolescence. There are several reasons for this: the adolescent is anxious because he is insecure; he is apt to have tensions of inferiority and rivalry as he struggles for recognition and as he hungers for approval. He has a desire to succeed and to win a place in society, but he is not entirely sure of his role. He is often subject to social pressures in order to learn faster than he naturally might. Parents correct him and blame him and chide him, and insist on his improvement; teachers assign to him certain requirements and judge him on the basis of his performance; his associates are apt to ridicule him, scorn him, spurn him, and make him feel uncomfortable and self-conscious. Religion adds to the burden of the other demands by appealing to him for obedience to Divine law, to measure up to high ethical and religious standards.

We might define guilt as the accusing sense of failure. It is both personal in the sense of accusing oneself and interpersonal in the sense of fearing that others will accuse. It is normal to seek and to miss goals, to strive and to fail — we, all of us, do it. Under stress, neurotic patterns may develop fears and projections of guilt.

Guilt is a problem that concerns religion first because religious people are responsible for fostering a sense of sin — talking and teaching of God as a stern judge, a watchful eye who is continually looking on and seeing even what we do in secret and what our secret thoughts may be, and teaching that God is an avenging and punishing Deity. High moral ideals, which are fostered by religion, increase tension and failure. Perfectionism is a painful stress that consistently brings on a sense of inferiority.

A theological professor of mine used to say, "In the light of the ideal, we all stand condemned." True as it is, that feeling of condemnation in the light of the ideal is a painful experience. Religion has also taught a vivid eschatology of reward and punishment in the future life to stimulate the urgency of attaining these ideals and the fear of falling short of them. Religious codes also have repressed sex and the lusts of the flesh with forbidding commandments —"Thou shalt not." They have added increasing emotional anxiety by cosmic imperatives which bring more urgency behind this sense of guilt.

Religious organizations and people, therefore, have a special responsibility because of fostering the sense of sin. We also have responsibility to provide a way of solving guilt problems. The burden becomes unbearable unless release is offered. Severe depressions and compulsions, withdrawal or paranoiac tendencies may arise in this way.

Psychiatrists seek to reduce guilt and relieve anxieties as one of their major objectives, while the clergy have induced and magnified the guilt. It may therefore appear that psychiatrists and religious leaders are working against each other, and each is apt to have mutual suspicion toward the other on the grounds of mistreating the deepest needs of life. The psychiatrist is accusing the clergy of adding unnecessarily to the burden of guilt and anxiety, while the clergy may feel that the psychiatrists are undermining the moral code and condoning what ought not to be condoned in order to reduce tension at the point of guilt. We must, therefore, meet this question fairly and squarely to maintain a healthy balance between apathy and overanxiety.

Without any anxiety at all, we have apathy, indifference, which is as serious a problem as overanxiety; and, at the other extreme, overanxiety induced by a sensitive conscience may bring distress and disturbances of personality. Therefore, we cannot rest content with either extreme. We must have conscientiousness enough without having overconscientiousness and anxiety. We need tension enough to work for progress, guilt feelings to promote striving, effort and growth; within bounds, we see that they are a healthy and normal experience. But we need also ways of release from the burden of guilt and relief from overanxieties about the trivial things, for the people who worry the most are apt to be worrying needlessly about trivialities and in this way disabling and crippling themselves from the largest usefulness and freedom.

Traditionally, we have developed religious services to meet the need of reducing anxiety. Repentance and an opportunity for change are offered to everyone by the teachings of our religious faith. We believe that whatever a person may have done, if he repents of it honestly, and earnestly desires to change his life, he may start anew. Also, we have provided for confession and catharsis of repressed emotions; the Roman Catholic Church has made a sacrament of confession and has invited every person to come regularly to the confessional for the releasing of these emotional repressions, while the Protestant clergymen and Jewish rabbis have made themselves available for pastoral counseling. They have had the doors of their offices open and have called frequently in the homes of their people and encouraged them in the releasing of repressed emotions through confession in informal ways.

Forgiveness and reparation are also encouraged by our religious traditions, teaching that God is not merely a God of wrath but that He is a God of love; that He is not merely a Divine, stern judge, but that He is also a for-

giving Father who understands the weakness of the flesh —
"He remembereth our frame and knoweth that we are dust"
— and therefore is willing and able to forgive us for our
failures and mistakes, and also to encourage us in making
good, righting wrongs, repairing damages, and becoming a
new creature.

My teaching of theological students may strike a bit
above the adolescent age, though I have been known to
say that persons are adolescents until they marry and until
they are in a full-time and satisfying vocation. Students
in theological school are not likely to have attained either
of those goals. They are in the inferior position that students are in, as schoolboys under teachers, and have not
attained the adjustments either of establishing themselves
as the head of a family or as the head of a church. So,
even if they may be twenty-two years of age, I think it is
interesting to consider from the standpoint of the adolescent problem of guilt what these theological students say
about sins.

In reply to my question, "What are my chief sins;
which are most prevalent and most serious?" these answers
are summarized. First, laziness and procrastination. "I
enjoy dreaming about doing something more than doing
it." "If I have failed to do my best, I have sinned." "If I
were not so lazy, I might be a power. Because I am lazy,
I don't organize well, and use the maze of things I face
as an excuse for all my failures." "Laziness keeps me from
doing my best."

Moral constantly comes in here, too. "Seeking lustful
interests — sex, intemperance in eating, neglecting sleep,
unwholesome thoughts, and unclean speech." I think there
is considerably less of this among theological students, yet
no human being is free entirely from this problem.

The third is jealousy; secret delight in doing better
than others; intolerance. "I cannot tolerate others doing

or believing what I do not." "Very seldom do I show jealousy, but down in my heart I find it difficult to be genuinely happy over someone else's success."

The fourth is indifference, pride, and self-righteousness; lack of sympathy for others; feelings of superiority; being too critical of others.

The fifth is selfishness; failing to help others in need, recognizing selfishness as a major source of trouble in the world, selfishness that one's whims be pleased, and thoughtlessness of others.

Sixth is hypocrisy. This covers a multitude of sins — bitterness toward one's fellow; continuance of sin despite the realization that it is a sin; "the sin of glossy, artful, capacity or willingness to cover up the grosser sins by excusing them or confessing the lesser ones," says one student.

Another student said, "My worst habit is reading in bed." (He is fortunate if that is his worst habit.) "Excusing myself from church work for school work that is never done." "It is easy to pretend to be something that I am not." "Teaching against the evils which I practice in my own life."

The seventh is mind-wandering and day-dreaming; lack of discipline and study in church work.

Eighth is dishonesty. "I like to stretch the truth in order to make a story a little more sensational with exaggerations and implications I know are false." "How I like to rationalize! I can almost always give logical reasons to justify evils I have done."

Ninth is lack of real devotion to God. "I hope to devote my life to Him. There is no positiveness to make it worthwhile." "Lack of religious coordination to the goal I have set. Tangents fly off in many directions."

"Why do I sin?" is the next question, and these are the answers, briefly:

The first is habits; the line of least resistance; day-dreaming as the substitute for doing. "I sin because I am inherently weak, prone to follow the line of least resistance." "I do not go around sinning on purpose; I don't get a kick out of sinning; most of my sins feel as though I'm helpless to meet the needs of the hour." "It's easier to sin than to do good." And another says, "Habits of thinking I have formed."

The second reason is desire. "I would almost rather go on sinning, yet I am most concerned not to."

Third, ignorance. "If not acquainted with all the facts of the situation, I will not act according to the facts." And another student says, "Because at the moment it seems the best thing to do."

Fourth, "Human nature is unmoral." "Tendencies toward good or evil desires are left to free choice." "Because I am not divine, I must struggle." "It is human imperfection — not born in sin, but to sin and also to goodness."

A fifth reason suggested childhood training or lack of discipline.

Sixth is "lack of faith in myself."

Then, I asked, "What are my chief worries and anxieties?" Here is a list of them:

The first one is success; perfection; progress. "My chief worry is that I shall fail as a minister in Christian life." "I worry about doing my work well."

The second answer is, "Everything — mostly myself. In worrying about myself, there is the dread that I could stagnate, drift into carelessness and unproductive work habits and thus become a burden to the cause I wish to serve." "I worry about what other people think of me." There is an intense desire to be well thought of.

A third answer is social relationships; conflicts and separations; family opposition and refusal to co-operate; stubborn selfishness. "I can meet folks easily, but beyond the speaking acquaintanceship, my relationship with others is often rather shallow. I have a shyness which often keeps me from feeling wholly at ease in a group who are having a good time. Moreover, when I have made a rich friendship, I often let it slide by, failing to follow up a correspondence or leaving a situation in a state of slight misunderstanding."

Fourth, "The question of my own ability — if only I could be sure of myself. If only I could know that I have the necessary qualifications." "If I were positive that I can do a worthwhile work, then I should become a more diligent worker." Another says, "I have a horror of becoming another stick of wood which has found its way into the Christian ministry."

Fifth, financial matters. "The salary is irregular, and there come times when there is very little between our home and starvation." "Anyone who has regard for human values must be anxious about what is going on in the world; there is a general unrest of troubled conditions. Shall I remain in school and prepare for either the chaplaincy or full-time pastorate, or should I quit school, resign the church, and enter some service that my conscience will accept?" (You will recognize that that was during the war.)

Sixth, world crises. "Worry for fear I am not doing all I could do in these moments; thoughts arise about joining the Army or Navy, or some such work. The work I am in is as important as any work if it is done well, and I must do it well, and worries will disappear."

Seventh. "The effectiveness of my church as a community agency. I want it to be the best church possible. When it doesn't live up to my expectations, when it fails, I worry about it. Its failure is a reflection on the effectiveness of my ministry."

Eighth, health and welfare of family and friends. "I

have already had five college friends killed in action, and this sorrow has increased my anxiety for others whom I know so well." Another worries about his father's health, about a brother's being drafted out of college; personal health worries as affecting vocation, marriage, efficiency, and happiness.

Ninth, the future. "I worry about the future; I wonder what it holds in store for me." "I think about what I might be doing ten years from now — many times it appears uncertain." "I worry about my vocation as it will work out and my possible effectiveness."

Another question was, "What am I doing to solve these problems?"

First, redirecting one's interests; that is, in management of one's thoughts, by governing the thinking process, one controls the issues that present themselves to the mind.

The second answer is, "In keeping busy, there is no time to worry. Occupation leaves little time for worry." "Devotion to the responsibility that is mine." "My antidote to worry is to cultivate an active unconcern."

Third, prayer and perspective; assurance of God's presence helps to cope with worry — "Feeling that God showed me what is to be done, as if God were right beside me and was trying to tell me he would be always with me and I need not worry about sermons or dealing intelligently with people, that all people needed would be coming from Him." Another — "By prayer, one is released from the nervous tensions that hinder the freedom of the spirit. Prayer opens the heart to God and lets assurance and peace pervade the mind."

Fourth, intelligently attacking the problem. "I think about what to do instead of actually doing it. To correct this, instead of thinking, I do something. The action may not be the best possible, but at least it accomplishes something instead of wasting time about what not to do. Some problems I can best meet by direct frontal attack on them."

Fifth is encouragement of friends. "Friends who know me best believe in me and tell me I will be a good minister. Their judgment should be worth something. I hear their opinions and fervently pray that they are right."

Sixth, development of serenity through prayer. "A calm retreat will help when we face difficulty. It can be found, however, that it is something that dwells within the mind over a long period of time and has its roots in the philosophy which we hold deeply imbedded in life and it will sustain us between so-called problems." Another says, "I cannot make life too carefree, but I meet it courageously and do not worry over my failures, but conquer them." "I can only do so much," says another, "only my best, and only for that am I responsible. I must not strive for the impossible ideal."

Seventh, employing tensions for achievement. "A certain amount of anxiety keeps me toned up to doing work according to schedule. Worry or anxiety in themselves are useless and inhibiting, and they both should be overcome, but worry with a purpose, or conscientious anxiety is productive of more intensive action — they are incentives, and, as such, are valuable." Another says, "I resolved tension by deciding whether there is anything which I could do about the matter. If there is nothing, I might as well resign myself to the outcome of events; if there is something which can be done, the best course of action must be decided upon, and the action ought to provide an outlet for worry." Another says, "I believe these anxieties are necessary if life is to be lived conscientiously and purposefully and fully. There is a need to know life, to have concern over the things we love and value lest we lose them."

The eighth is better understanding. "I believe that truth is the solution to the whole problem of united Christianity as fundamentalism clashes with modernism."

"Earnest study, especially of the Bible." Another —"God is working through the tension of anxiety to stimulate me to achieve progress and growth."

A ninth answer is religious faith. "I believe that the practice of my religious faith should remove and overcome these problems." "Some problems cannot be taken to others, but only to God. Here I feel a real comradeship with the Divine, and it is the greatest of all help, for it is through God that ultimately all problems are solved, all worries and anxieties overcome." And another says, "God is for me — adding His desire, His strength, to mine."

This brings something of the fresh air of personal experience into our discussion of these guilt and anxiety problems of the adolescent.

In conclusion, I should like to ask, "What can religion do for the adolescent?" First, accept him on growing terms. Religious organizations, the church or synagogue, have steps of approval for every major stage in growing life: Baptism for the infant; confirmation; or joining the church on preparatory and full membership for the adolescent; marriage to solemnize another stage of development; also recognition in the vocational life, major crises, and at the time of death.

It's very important that adolescents feel accepted and approved. They are sensitive to disapproval and they get a lot of criticism — well-meaning criticism, but too much of it. So, accepting the adolescent on growing terms means accepting him for what he is at this age, and expecting him to grow up to the next stage beyond. Church membership does give approval and a sense of belonging to a group.

We need to offer more permissive relationships to adolescents with less scolding and less condemning, more appreciation and recognition of the good that he does. We must expect growth of the adolescent and give him adult roles, because without adult roles, we keep him childish; but with adult roles, responsibilities and respect, he responds and measures up to what we expect of him

A second thing that religion can do for the adolescent is to provide group activity and therapy. Youth fellowships offer boy-girl associations in his own age groups. These are very important, and along with them should come sex education and honesty in considering the intimate things of life.

Nowhere in our society is sex education adequately conducted. The school neglects it; the parents are afraid to touch it, most of them; and the church does little about it. However, it does appear that the church is doing more than any other agency in society, and it also appears that in the group is the best opportunity for sex education. It isn't so embarrassing as in face to face — I mean one to one relationships — and I am in favor also of coeducational sex education. It is good for boys and girls to hear these things said in the presence of each other. They have a common knowledge, then, to understand, to live up to. It also helps them to release their embarrassment, this self-consciousness in relation to each other, if we can talk out loud in their presence about sex and they can talk out loud about it in the presence of the other sex.

The group activities also provide spontaneity — spontaneity to act, to speak, to play, to worship, and to serve at their level of development in co-operation with others of their own age group. There is need for more democratic participation and leadership. We are rather dictatorial in the home, the school, and the church. We need to practice the democracy that we preach and give young people more leadership, more freedom for the expression of their growing sense of responsibility.

A third thing that religion can do for the adolescent is to forgive his mistakes and failures. We can avoid religious perfectionist demands, for they are fatal to peace of mind. We can note the signs of guilt and anxiety, compunctions, punishments invited, which show that the problem of guilt is being wrestled with. We need to detect these subtle signals of guilt in the adolescent, and then, with good humor and perspective, to prevent his and our taking failures too seriously. It is his right to make mistakes and to learn by them, and he will learn better by them if we do not magnify his mistakes or the feeling of guilt for them.

Also, the teaching of divine forgiveness and the giving of absolution with the opportunity for a new start are important — "Neither do I condemn thee; go and sin no more." This is a good balance, it refuses to condemn and thus relieves guilt. "Go and sin no more" offers an opportunity for a new start and freedom from the incumbrance of former guilt feelings.

A fourth thing that religion can do for the adolescent is to release his emotional responses creatively. There are cathartic values in worship, confession, and discussion. We need to help adolescents channel their emotions to constructive uses, making love, vocation, all the relationships of life, dealing with the grief situations that adolescents often face in the loss of parents or friends, and dealing with them cathartically rather than repressively, bringing the ministry of religion to a dignity and a sense of comradeship at such times. Then, we need to sublimate their basic drives to spiritual expressions, not to stamp them out or deny them, but to elevate them to a socially acceptable spiritual expression. There are many ways in which our basic drives for sex and ego can be expressed acceptably in our society, and we must help children and young people make a good bargain between the biological needs and the social standards of acceptance, helping them to find ways to express themselves successfully in ways that can be approved socially.

A fifth and final thing religion can do for the adolescent is to awaken his affections and extend his loyalties. To love and to be loved deeply and joyously is the right of every child, adolescent, and adult. We need to do more of it and encourage more of it than a stern puritanism or the careless indifference of our age usually permits. To identify self with others, to give thoroughgoing devotion to a cause, to learn its purposes, to live long in faithfulness, to discover social adventures of unselfish heroic deeds, larger achievements and satisfactions — in these ways, religion can do much for the adolescent in helping him to cope with his problems of guilt, to win larger achievements and larger joys in his attainments.

General Discussion

QUESTION: In the light of present psychiatric tendencies I wonder if Dr. Johnson could have assured those adolescent students that the nine points which he enumerated were not sins at all.

DR. JOHNSON: Sin is a theological concept which means disobedience to the will of God, and sins are usually classified as witting or unwitting, or sometimes minor and major, sins. It appears to me that many of these are minor sins. They are not crude or gross sins that are often characteristic of people in our age, but I suggest that, as we eliminate the grosser sins, we are apt to have remaining these refinements of sin. The tendency to procrastinate need not be called a sin, and yet if one has no guilt at all about it, he may waste time the rest of his life without the least concern, and thus not be as efficient and productive as he might be otherwise. I think laziness is a rather comfortable and not too serious predicament if it is intermittent, but if it is constant, laziness becomes a threat to the achievement of the values of which his life would be capable. So I feel that any sin or failure, as I have defined guilt as the accusative sense of failure, any vital failure may be a problem. First, if it's neglected entirely, it may lead to an increasing sense of failure; if it's given too much attention, with an overanxious conscience, it may become a neurotic tendency to worry about trifles.

That's why I say we need to strike a balance between apathy on the one hand, which is characteristic of the psychopath, and overanxiety on the other hand, which is characteristic of the neurotic.

QUESTION: There are many things in life which young people cannot define as good or bad, for there are some things which a Christian young man may do and not consider sinful, while a Jewish person doing the very same thing may consider it a sin. A Catholic young man may consider it sinful not to attend church on Sunday, and many a Protestant young man may have no qualms about it.

DR. JOHNSON: Well, we have varying conceptions of sin because sin is a human invention. It is our interpretation of what God wants us to do and wherein we fail to do God's will. As we progress ethically and religiously, we should move from the insignificant and trivial sins and feelings of guilt about the incidental and trivial faults up to a concern for the major moral questions of our time. We are in need of being more aware and more concerned about those who are starving, dispossessed; those who are discriminated against in an unjust social order; about the tendencies that make for war and competitive hatred and destruction. We need to focus our attention upon social sins, whereas, in the past and in the present, we may waste a lot of energy worrying about personal sins that are trivial.

So, it is our business to educate the conscience. We cannot expect a conscience to be healthy unless it is well educated, and it is for us to do a better job at educating our consciences at the points of what is more urgently significant in terms of human success and failure.

QUESTION: Don't we arrive at a fundamental dichotomy between the demands of psychiatry which, as I understand it, is concerned with the disabling tendencies in life, and those of religion which set up a man-made system of ethical beliefs.

DR. JOHNSON: Yes, we do, unfortunately. Religion has been too dependent upon traditions that are destructive in character, that is, they are deduced from premises which may not be true; while psychiatry has been more inductive, approaching the question from the standpoint of human experience and welfare rather than from abstract or traditional theological concepts. If I do injustice to either profession, I hope you will correct me. As I am of the theological profession, I am trying very hard to be honest with myself about theological tradition, and I say that I believe that theological traditions are deduced from premises which may not be true always. Psychiatrists probably have their deductive traditions, but I am not well acquainted with them. It appears that the psychiatrist is dealing with human needs in the personality before him, and that is what the minister should do. The clergyman should also start with human life and the needs of human life, and try to interpret God's will in terms of practical human situations.

QUESTION: Our attention has been directed to the fact that the adolescent mind is confused and often threatened as a result of many superstitions and guilt notions with regard to sex.

Dr. Johnson suggested that there were many things that organized religion might do to alleviate the situation. I wonder if Dr. Johnson would care to comment more concretely on what we might do, within the framework of organized religion, to help the adolescent come to a truer understanding of the problem of sex. Would he like to suggest some kind of preliminary curriculum for a group of adolescent boys such as might be found within any synagogue or church?

DR. JOHNSON: I would suggest beginning, first, with parents, young parents, who may not yet have babies or who are on the way to having them. If a pastor or a well-educated teacher can lead a club of young parents and go into the basic sex education for them and for growing children, it might be possible for these parents to answer the questions of children in their natural curiosity, one at a time, as they arise, which is the best way to do it if they can withdraw the excess emotion from the consideration of these matters. There should be more tolerance, more flexibility at that point.

To properly tell a boy and girl what they need to know takes a very skilful person. It takes a very skilful person to give sex education to a child in grade school, but surely it can be done, and I think that it might best be carried on in the regular classes of the church school as a part of the curriculum, lest it have too much hushed mystery and awe about it if they are set apart in some special place and room (in whispers) "to talk about sex."

Then we come to the adolescent age. As I have said, I believe that boys and girls of the adolescent age should study about sex together, and this can best be done, I think, in group fellowships. At the age of fifteen or sixteen, boy and girl relationships is the most popular topic for young people of that age. In many of our youth groups, that course is introduced for six weeks, perhaps, in which a discussion of boy and girl relationships is carried out at their level. Questions come about social dating, about petting, and about the various etiquettes and responsibilities in their new age, about problems in appreciating each other and going out together in couples.

Around the age of seventeen or eighteen, there is an interest in falling in love and becoming engaged. At this time a course is needed in the question of falling in love, or adventures in love (which is perhaps a little too exciting). This course, or one a little later, should deal with looking toward marriage or thinking about marriage.

Approaching the age of engagement, it has been my privilege, with my wife, to conduct courses at a Protestant church for this age group: first, the falling-in-love age, about sixteen, and second, the engagement group, young couples who formed together into a class because either they are engaged or they are "going steady" and thinking about it. There you can go into the specific questions of how to choose a mate, what are the qualities to look for that are most important, how to prepare for marriage, and think through these questions of the psychological adjustments of personalities to each other in the courtship age.

When we come to the question of marriage itself, there are economic questions of how to support a wife while you are in school, if that is the problem, or on a small income; questions of having children and of the sex relationships within marriage (which certainly need to be discussed before marriage). And then there is an opportunity for premarital counseling in which, when a young couple comes to talk about marriage, you can go into a question of the fears and apprehensions and uncertainties, and the problems and the things which need to be faced emotionally.

Likewise, at the time of marriage, the pastor is very close to the couple and to the families as they work their way through this exciting event. After marriage, there is the need for follow-up work, marital counseling. With pregnancy, there is the need for counseling again and free discussion of the emotional problems and adjustments to make. At this time and at the time of childbirth, of course, there is special recognition and christening and so on.

I have sought to suggest that, starting with the young couples who are going to have children and carrying through to the marriages of these children, there is constant need for an open honesty and consideration together of these matters, in groups and in individual counseling.

CHAPTER NINE

MARRIAGE

F. Alexander Magoun and Joseph Michaels

SECTION I — *F. Alexander Magoun*

Society says that marriage is a legal question. State legislatures, through laws and the courts, lay down certain qualifications to be fulfilled before people can marry, such as the necessity for a license, the achievement of a minimum age, a witnessed ceremony conducted by a legally qualified person, no other marriage already in existence, no close blood relationship between bride and groom (in many states first cousins cannot marry). These requirements are important, but they are only superficial.

Marriage is a many-sided relationship between a man and a woman, intended in our culture to continue until interrupted by death; the legal, social, economic, religious, and emotional aspects of which provide — theoretically at least — the best circumstances under which to conceive and to rear children; at the same time, offering the maximum opportunity for the greatest number of adults to live well rounded, happy lives as individuals.

There are many ways of being married. One can be married physically, or financially, or intellectually, or emotionally, as well as legally. In the ideal situation, wedlock includes bonds in all these areas. Unhappy indeed is the couple where the bond is only legal. "What God hath joined," expresses an unwarranted assumption which would surely be characterized as such by omniscient

NOTE: This material has been taken from Professor Magoun's book, *Courtship, Love and Marriage,* published by Harper and Brothers, New York, 1948.

wisdom. The idea that an agreement and a legal bond automatically confer happiness, because marriages are made in heaven by some mysterious and divine predestination, is sentimental tommyrot. If marriages are made in heaven, why do so many married people live in hell?

The basic forces which enter into the successful establishment and functioning of a marriage are many and varied. Marriage is fundamentally a problem of living happily together; a man and a woman united in the achievement of common goals to which they give their hopes, their thoughts, and their best efforts. They are two parts of the same team, with interlocking functions, and interdependent powers which will lead to quarreling unless successfully inter-related.

Marriage is essentially an adjustment between a man and a woman who are happy or unhappy because of what they are. Success or failure is largely in terms of the ability to interweave interests. Sharing the affection of a good-bye kiss in the morning; quiet enjoyment of a loving embrace at the evening homecoming, so that each feels this is the moment the other has been waiting for all day, and now his life is complete and overflowing once more; darting little affectionate glances at each other while sharing the day's experiences; sitting together in the lamplight in wordless understanding: these are the pattern into which marriage should be woven, but the threads must be held together by the strands of love.

Without realizing it, many people have an emotional attitude toward marriage akin to, "Now I shall have again the protection I enjoyed as a little child." It is true that a happy family is the highest of all sources of emotional security. It is true that marriage is the best method for a well balanced person to effect emotional completion. It is true that we do not live by bread alone; with it we need companionship, laughter, mutuality of value standards.

But so many brides and grooms expect a marriage to provide solutions for all the difficult struggles within their personalities. So many assume that it will no longer be necessary for them to stand on their own feet because now they are to have sanctuary, and happiness will follow safety.

Marriage provides a new atmosphere, but both husband and wife meet the same old problems of life, as well as some new ones — and do it with the same old behavior techniques. Each now has a new title role, but the parts assigned them by their parents during childhood have so typed their acting that each will play almost the same character as before. If they have the emotional maturity to be able to accept personal responsibilities, they will create together a healthy atmosphere in which both individuals will flourish and develop even more inner strength with which to meet problems. If they are not emotionally mature, if their integrity is not complete, if there is not true internal consistency in their personalities the resulting inner conflicts will produce an unhealthy atmosphere in which each individual will frustrate the other, thus denying both an opportunity for spontaneous self-expression.

Far too many young people approach marriage with a romantic and egocentric attitude, full of daydreams which are concerned with *getting*, never with *giving*. They have not progressed emotionally beyond the "gimme" stage. Such an attitude is not only wishful thinking, it is turning the church aisle into a warpath. Here the desire for a happy home is only a desire for the benefits of a happy home, not a readiness to accept the responsibility and the work of producing the necessary conditions to create a happy home. This is expecting too much of marriage. Of course it leads to bitter disillusionment. Daydreaming of the end result, with no regard for means, is only silly sentimentalism.

Daydreams about marriage often have to do with:
(1) escape from an unhappy environment
(2) sexual satisfaction
(3) devoted "mothering" (for the man)
(4) economic security and social status (for the woman)

Under these conditions, it is not the reality of Barbara that Albert is marrying, but a fantasy Albert has pictured. Nevertheless, she can only be herself, as he will surely find out sooner or later. Then come bewilderment, disappointment, anger. He thought Barbara was a goddess, and behold, she is only a human being, afraid of mice and thunderstorms, wanting to spend money for things which seem to him inconsequential, running the house in ways that backslide from the true faith exemplified by his mother, simmering in resentment on occasion, objecting to his habit of reading the paper at the breakfast table, telling him the neighborhood gossip but turning on the radio when he starts to talk about the office. It is a great shock to waken to this reality and to discover that marriage is not what he thought it would be. There is cruel tragedy in it. But the trouble is not with marriage; the trouble is with a civilization which permits, and to some degree encourages, the stupidity of believing happy marriage is given us like a Christmas present. Why think of marriage only in terms of happiness? No one approaches a profession that way. Happiness is not a right we possess, it must be earned, and as always, the best rewards come after years of effort.

What is love? The questions concerning its nature have been as persistent as the yearning to possess it. "I can't bother with a definition, but everybody knows what love is," only covers an unwillingness to recognize ignorance. The more accurately a thing is understood the more readily it can be defined. Without a clear concept of what

love is, how can anyone approach marriage intelligently?
Much that is labeled love has nothing to do with love.
Indeed, part of it is hate. We have made love a hopelessly
ambiguous word. "I love lobster thermidor." "Don't you
just love that hat!" "If you love me, you will do this for
me." "Her death was such a tragedy. They were deeply
in love." Obviously the gourmet, the milliner, the domineering parent, and the old acquaintance mean very different things when they say "love."

*Love is the passionate[1] desire on the part of two or
more people to produce together the conditions under
which each can spontaneously express his real self; to
produce together an intellectual soil and an emotional
climate in which each can flourish, far superior to what
either could achieve alone.* It is an intimate relatedness
based on the mutual approval and affirmation of the character and integrity of the personalities involved. It is not
a situation where two partners think more of each other
than they do of themselves. It is a situation where two
partners think more of the partnership than they do of
themselves. It is an interweaving of interests and a facing
of sacrifice[2] together for the sake of both. It is the feeling
of security and contentment that comes with the adequate
satisfaction of each person's emotional needs through their
mutual efforts. It is man's superlative method of self-
realization and survival.

Love is feeling, and much of feeling cannot be ex-

---

[1] Passion is being in the grip of an emotional experience so big that it
possesses you, and you can do nothing about it, like the feelings which
possess a person in the presence of birth, or death, or love.

[2] Sacrifice comes from two Latin words, *sacra* and *ficio*, meaning "to
make holy." Thus, an individual gives up something highly desirable to
him for the sake of protecting, of developing but especially of improving a
person, end, or ideal dearer to him than the thing given up. Sacrifice
usually involves self-denial, but it has no implication, as is commonly
supposed, of being exploited, dominated, imposed upon, or victimized.

pressed in words. To say, "I love you," is not necessarily to love. The word is not the thing. Words are puny; feelings are powerful. Words are only the trivia that convey ideas — usually somebody else's ideas. Feeling is life itself, and fullness of life depends upon breadth, and depth, and reality of feeling. It is relatively easy to share ideas. Many emotions are extremely difficult to share. Nevertheless, love is impossible until one can *feel* differences and similarities in people, and feel a respect for them.

Most of us do not correctly feel what is going on within ourselves or within anyone else. What we feel is convention and social obligation because we were brought up that way for fear we would obey our impulses. To know what one is feeling does not mean that it will be expressed impulsively. It is then even easier to wait until one knows how he wants to express it. As a matter of fact, the breaking through of impulse is proof of repressed feelings. There is no explosion unless first some force has been imprisoned.

Nothing can be truly known until it has been experienced and assimilated on the level of feeling. To know what one wants and needs, requires first an understanding of what one's feelings are. What is one's fundamental nature? What is one seeking to express in living his particular life in his particular environment? Of the great variety of emotional impulses which continuously come to everyone, and which no one can avoid, which does one genuinely desire to develop and to express for his own best long-run satisfaction? To discover one's self is to discover what human nature is like, and therefore, to have an understanding of what people are like and the purposes for which they were created — including the need to love and to be loved.

Love between two people who cannot sense and share each other's emotions is impossible. Though they may be devoted and actively loyal to each other, they cannot be in love. To love is to feel with fidelity to the facts, and thus to know what each wants and needs in order to produce together the conditions under which each can grow into his real self.

Loving behavior is natural wherever a person can be his real self without pretense. There is no other way to be free from the conflicts and the repressions which destroy the spontaneous, creative self-expression which underlies love. *The more completely one can express his real self to another person, the more deeply he can love.*

Love carries through the whole gamut of emotions, producing a kinship of body, mind, and spirit. It is not an occasional tingling with anticipation. It is not the idealistic, emotionally dishonest, self-denial which proclaims that the essence of love and morality is the subordination of one's individual satisfactions to the service of someone else. This is self-abdication, and where there is someone surrendering himself, there is also someone collecting the offering. Such a relationship is closer to slavery than to love.

Thus two people can only love each other when they naturally and honestly fulfill each other's emotional needs. There must be a mutuality to loving behavior. The satisfaction-seeking efforts of each must, to a large extent, provide simultaneous satisfaction for the other. This is why love intensifies and grows deeper with time, not by domination or submission, but by mutual development; two people singing to one music, sometimes in unison, sometimes in parallel harmonic intervals, sometimes in pleasing counterpoint, sometimes in acceptable dissonances . . . but always at least two, and always together.

When we react to stimuli which concern other people's needs, it is because at the same time our needs are involved in some direct or indirect way. So our own happiness is a prerequisite for making other people happy. Happiness is to be found in forgetting one's self? By no means. The alcoholic, the psychotic, the drug addict are all seeking self-forgetfulness. The only road to complete self-forgetfulness is suicide. Happiness comes through giving one's self, freely and completely, to an emotionally satisfying cause.

There are many false emotions which mislead us and impose upon us, the most dangerous of which, at the outset, look like love. All of them are difficult to recognize at first; most of them are brutually unmasked by time. Among them are: mistaking romance—which stresses glamour and adventure rather than character—for love; a parasitic dependence upon another person because of being too weak or too afraid to stand alone; sexual desire aroused by physical beauty or perhaps sheer energy and zest for life; need to exploit someone to gain self-assurance through money, prestige, power; living life vicariously through another person because of inability to be one's self; a compulsive desire to feel needed; a man intent upon the conquest of a woman to mother him; a woman determined not to be an old maid, or in search of a meal ticket; either or both craving the rapturous feeling of reassurance which comes when an individual is treated as though he were in fact that which in his glorified fantasies about himself he believes himself to be. Naturally the greater the discrepancy between the fantasy and reality, the greater the need for outside reassurance of its reality. The greater the reassurance, the bigger the thrill of feeling "I am lovable after all,". . . until reality brings the deception to an end, as it always does, in the headache of the morning after.

Each one of the counterfeits is based on some kind of self-centered, irrational reassurance. In no one of them— no matter how one may temporarily fool himself to the contrary—is there a sincere, consuming desire to produce *with the other person* the conditions under which *each* can be and spontaneously express his real self. In no one of them is there a sincere desire to produce together an intellectual soil and an emotional climate in which *each* can flourish, far superior to what either could achieve alone. To fail in this is to fall short of love.

We think we are in love because of the way another person makes us feel. This is a desire for the emotions created in us by the other individual *at the moment;* it is not loving him. Love is not a method for keeping a person happy about himself: that is infatuation. It knows not the underlying fear and uncertainty of the reassurance-seeking swain who hugs passionately and whispers, "You do love me, darling, don't you? You know you do." Love is not delight in *me,* love is self-realization together in *us.* Two mutually infatuated people can want each other desperately without love, and without sensing the emotional insincerity which consumes them during the delicious and palpitant intimacy of necking in a taxi. Neither realizes how allergic he is to himself; neither perceives he is experiencing little more than a cheap reassurance. What seems to be love is but blind delight in being treated as though one were perfection itself, when actually one is dissatisfied with one's self.

Hate often masquerades as love. The woman driving a man by nagging or insinuation into a profession for which he has little inclination, "Because I'm thinking of your best good, dear," is trying to destroy a part — or the whole — of him in the hope of getting in exchange more money, or more freedom, or more social prestige for herself. The self-righteous father, luring or compelling his son into study in a field for which the boy has no interest, is a destroyer. The husband and wife, continually attacking each other in such words as, "The trouble with you is ...," are bent on emotional murder.

Hate develops from a continuing state of repressed anger over fears we refuse to recognize. Like a boil, it is an attempt to concentrate an emotional infection, and to throw it out of the system. It is the symptom of something wrong, and it is also the attempt to get well.

No two human beings can possibly live together in the most intimate emotional relationship known to man without sometimes frustrating each other. When love is blocked it turns to anger and hate. But change the situation a little, remove the frustration, and affection pours out once more. Then comes the sweetness of making up after a quarrel. Nevertheless, the Fates should not be tempted by allowing this to happen often. Calmer ways of meeting frustration need to be developed.

If the marriage is worth much, both partners will become happier, more emotionally mature, more self-confident and spontaneous; but this is impossible unless they have the right raw materials to start with, a knowledge of sound principles of human relations and good methods of applying them, and the vision of attainable objectives sincerely desired by both. Such developments are not random and confused, but planned and purposeful. Marriage cannot be expected to run itself by wishful thinking. The interlocking leadership and the interweaving responsibilities of husband and wife must be constructive, and this constructive action is part of a thought-out, adequate process.

Husband and wife must enter the marriage with honest unity of purpose. The more things they care about in common, the closer together they will be in mind and emotion. This does not mean that husband and wife cannot have special and private interests of their own. It does mean that there cannot be a major conflict of those responses to life, which determine our standard of values, for the atmosphere of the home is determined by the interweaving of the self-expression and the self-evaluation of its members. Mere agreement is not to be confused with emotional unity. There can be agreement despite loss of emotional unity, as when someone tilts his nose at angle *theta* with a now-she-sees-I'm-right air of virtue. And there can be disagreement with no loss of emotional unity, as when husband and wife sincerely seek to explain to each other their respective positions, with no attempted coercion.

As for responsibilities and authorities, husband and wife play many different and mutually overlapping parts — a worker here, the purchasing agent there, both worker and executive somewhere else, clear lines of responsibility for this, no lines of authority for that. So many confused and interlocking parts, all involved in each other, make an organization chart on paper practically impossible, to say nothing of anything which could be nailed down in practice. But marriage can be made to work if husband and wife have a good sense of administration and are sincerely motivated by a desire for togetherness. Like a watch, the marriage works because of the right relationship of its parts, not just because the parts are there.

The family is an organization in which two sexes, and often two or more generations at a time, face this problem of relatedness in the creation of a common atmosphere. They exercise influence upon each other, varying from outright force, through calculated persuasion, to a spontaneous effort to find the truth together. They consciously and subconsciously impose difficulties upon one another. They invent outlets for individual self-expression. They undertake a wide variety of responsibilities.

The only valid basis for the existence of any organization — family, factory, or nation — is to create a mutually desired final result in terms of the co-ordinated action of its members toward their objective. This means:

(1) Co-ordinated desires: shared planning, on appropriate levels, of what the objectives ought to be.

(2) Co-ordinated decisions: settlement, again on appropriate levels of what, where, when, how, by whom the job is to be done.

(3) Co-ordinated action: each doing his job at the right time in the right way.

Under these circumstances, the operation of the family would result from an interflow of ideas, attitudes, problems, and mutually-arrived-at solutions which integrate them into the most reasonable and effective action *over the long run.*

This is co-operation. This is an emotionally secure relationship, not a threatening or frustrating one. This is respect for personalities and personality differences, so that each individual can work in the area of his aptitudes. This is equal concern for one's own legitimate interests and the further needs and desires of the others. This is properly relating people because it first distinguishes between their abilities, weaknesses, wants. This is achieving unity because it recognizes that the whole consists of separate and distinct parts which must be correctly related. This is mutual help, mutal encouragement, continual adjustment on each level of experience, stemming from — and in turn re-creating — right emotional relationships.

The solution of family disagreement and the ability to co-ordinate decisions depend, for one thing, upon the existence of a background of confidence in each other; a sort of generalized emotional security reservoir. How convinced is each person that he can discuss disagreements sincerely, revealing without hesitation just what he feels, thinks, sees? No pretense, no exaggeration, no insincerity; just complete trust and genuineness. How assured is he that in spite of differences of opinion, the others accept him for his real self, believe in him, wholeheartedly want the marriage and the home? How certain can he be that this is not an "all or none" relationship? How genuinely does his conduct make the others feel he wants to build depth as well as length and breadth into their lives by contributing his share in the establishment of these conditions? In a crisis will he undertake more than his usual share?

If he does not want these conditions, the only way he can be brought to want them is through some crisis which leads (not compels) him to see the evil results on himself of his desire to take advantage of or to exert power over those he thinks he loves. He is, in reality, trying to imprison and then to devour their lives. People can nourish each other, physically and emotionally, but they cannot long feed on each other.

A continuing stream of confidence, swelling into a reservoir, provides a reserve of trust and faith in each other by which to deal with actual or anticipated frustrations, and helps to meet them more calmly and realistically. It is a basis of accepting each other which transcends the misunderstanding of the moment. It provides assurance to each person that even though desires clash, decisions will not be final until they provide for everyone's legitimate needs in so far as is reasonably possible. It will not be done by taking a vote. Ballots show how people are divided, not where they agree. It will be done by patiently working toward a unifying "sense of the meeting," as the Quakers do.

In order to build such a reservoir of confidence and security, husband and wife must bring to the marriage or go through the agonizing pain of developing:

(1) Emotional maturity.
(2) Mutual compatibility in fundamental standards of what is important and worth-while, so that specific evaluations will be seen as only specific, and therefore, not the "be-all" and the "end-all."

(3) Empathy, with which to *feel* each other's emotional responses.

(4) Absence of undue irritation or interference from outside sources — in-laws, for example.

The security reservoir must be filled from streams of confidence welling up in many areas of the marriage. This is not a static thing. Like water, it will evaporate unless replenished. It can be drained by domination, or hiding resentment under cynicism, or camouflaging with false independence a need for loving and being loved, or even by excessive self-sacrifice. In what direction behavior will then turn is probably governed largely by generalized emotional attitudes.

When heavy demands have been made upon the supply, the reservoir must be quickly replenished, for feelings of insecurity spread from one area to another faster and more powerfully than do feelings of confidence. We can always destroy more swiftly than we can create.

When the reservoir fills faster than it empties, love grows, until at last even the casual observer perceives that the marriage has patience, love, and strength in reserve when decisions are difficult to co-ordinate.

Succesful marriage is a creative achievement. It does not come just because of a romantic thrill. It is not to be had by reaching out for a marriage license as one would pluck a lovely flower. It comes only with specialized knowledge and hard work.

There is no human situation in which all problems have been solved. It is fantasy to think there is, or can be, perfect harmony in marriage. Differences are always present, and they matter. But they can usually be solved by facing them honestly, understanding them, and wanting to work them out. Differences can even be fruitful, as the glorious blending of a variety of tone and timbre demonstrates when a great orchestra raises its voices with common intention. When there is no unity of purpose and each musician goes his own independent way, the result is only noise. The oboe may be more plaintive and penetrating, the violin more brilliant, but whether the oboe is superior or inferior to the violin is entirely beside the point. What matters is that each instrument play its own part well, and that the result is far superior to what any instrument could produce alone.

What matters is that each member of the family plays his part well, and that the result is far superior to what any individual could produce alone. Whether father or mother is superior to junior is entirely beside the point. Only a little child can bring a certain ring of laughter to the household; only an old person can contribute a certain unshakable tranquility; and the only way for any member of the family to have something — junior included — is to share it.

We rub shoulders with the thousands; we can share our hearts with few. But there is no substitute for love, just as there is no substitute for sex, and no substitute for marriage. The need for love is as universal as the need for bread. Without it, men seek money, or power, or fame, or a succession of physically beautiful women — poor, impoverished, starved souls seeking to benumb their loneliness by picking up shiny, frosted crumbs under the table of life. Few of them face stark reality as Turgenev did when he said, "I would give up my fame and all my art if there were one woman who would care whether I came home late for dinner."

It is not possible to live much of a life alone, for to live alone is to half live. To live selfishly is to fear living. To love, is to live two lives, one's own and that of the beloved. All of us need other people. But when two people use each other chiefly for compulsive reassurance, the result is exploitation. Any selfish motive is destructive even to a friendly relationship. For love, each must be willing to give fully and freely of himself, and to accept the other for what he is, not for what he can give. This is only possible where both are so emotionally mature and so close together in their attitude toward life, that deviations by either from behavior expected or desired by the other will almost never be felt as a threat to the personality of the other.

When a machine, an organization, or a family fails to respond adequately with replacements or sound new sections for worn out parts, breakdown is coming. There may be temporary rallies, but the end is near. It does not take long for the new-found intimacy of the honeymoon to metamorphose into the reality of everyday living: novelty gives way to routine, and unless steps are taken, stagnation will set in.

There are price tags on a happy marriage, and few bargains. A good marriage builds memories to cherish and cherishes them, for the great achievement in life is not money, or power, or fame, but a truly happy home.

Section II — *Joseph Michaels*

Prior to the war, there was one divorce out of every six marriages in the United States; in 1945 there was one divorce out of every four marriages. During the first four years of marriage, 36 per cent of divorces are granted and during the first nine years of marriage, 66 per cent of divorces occur; so that it can readily be seen that the period of the first ten years of marriage is the most vulnerable time as far as divorce is concerned.

During critical periods such as war, there are factors which strengthen and weaken the cohesive forces in society and in the individual. The increase in delinquency and divorce may be the results of the weakening process. In peacetime there is greater opportunity and more time for each partner to learn to know the other, and decisions can be reached which are tempered by mature reflection. War, in its acceleration of all reactions, leads to hasty marriages, enforced separations, and interferes with the healthy development of a stable family unit. The saying in peacetime of "Marry in haste, repeat or repent at leisure," becomes even more true in war time.

One of the positive contributions of the war was a fuller recognition of psychiatry and its diffuse permeation into all spheres of life. It is of interest that the realistic aspects of human problems are reflected in the publication of two novels by the same author, Charles Jackson. As you know, *The Lost Weekend,* deals with problems of the alcoholic, and his most recent book, *The Fall of Valor,* is a study of the death of a marriage. It is no accident that representatives from the field of religion have become concerned with psychiatric and social problems. The recent book of Rabbi Liebman, *Peace of Mind,* attempts to consummate a marriage of psychiatry and religion. Rabbi Goldstein, out of a vast experience with marital problems has written a book, *Marriage and Family Counseling,*[1] which I would like to recommend to all of you. Rabbi Goldstein presents five factors which may be useful in evaluating a marital problem:

(1) The legal implications of marriage in which rights and certain responsibilities are involved, especially the greater number of privileges which women now enjoy.

(2) Economic: the question of adequate income; the postponement of having children because of financial stress.

(3) Biological: blood tests, physical examinations. In short, the health of the prospective partners.

---

[1] Goldstein, S. E., *Marriage and Family Counseling.* New York: McGraw-Hill Book Co., 1945.

(4) Psychological: the suitability of the temperament of each partner and their knowledge of each other.

(5) Ethical ideals which pertain to the code of conduct.

On my return from military service, the first case (which we shall call the family of Mrs. A) referred to me by a family service agency consisted of the following problems: constant marital friction, frequent separations, a drinking husband, the family dependent on Department of Public Welfare, and a child who is a behavior problem. This is a typical and frequent problem encountered in social service agencies. It is presented from a sociologic and psychologic point of view and my summary is abstracted from the summary which the agency prepared. The agency wanted to know whether anything could be done to help the mother attain a greater maturity in her relation to the family. How much capacity for constructive relationship does the mother appear to have? Can she be expected, with help, to give the child more security than at present? Although the agency had had contact with the mother off and on in the past, in which she was assisted in obtaining housework, in November, 1945, her health became poor and she could not keep her job. She was generally upset and frequently came to the agency for advice. There had been several separations and reconciliations with her husband. The limited funds of the agency necessitated obtaining additional financial aid from the Department of Public Welfare. The mother was in her early thirties but looked close to forty. She was rather unattractive in appearance and had a somewhat combative manner.

Her mother died when she was very young and she was brought up by her grandmother. Her relatives had all disapproved of her mother's marriage and had considered her father of "no account trash." He was promiscuous, a drunkard, offered little support, never accepted responsibility, and was abusive to the mother. During the childhood of Mrs. A, she always yearned to be with her father and in adolescence she ran away to live with him and his mistress for a short period. Although she was resentful of her father's abuse and neglect, she hoped that he might love her and care for her despite the contrary evidence.

Mrs. A left high school before finishing and had done housework and worked as a waitress. When she was eighteen, she had an affair with a married man and became pregnant — the child in question was the offspring of this affair. Since then she had numerous affairs with other men: she lived for five years with a married man who was separated from his wife but not divorced. Later she became interested in her present husband who was attached to another woman, and following the birth of her second child, she brought him to court on a support charge and later he married her. During their marriage he never supported her adequately, and drank constantly. They quarrelled frequently, and there were many separations for short periods, in which Mrs. A would take the initiative, telling him that he could get out and find a room. She felt that he did not really love her or the child, in spite of the fact that he had been dependently devoted to her and she complained about his excessive sexual demands. It seemed that every time he was about to become successful or more adequate, she would begin to nag him as if to punish him, so that she alternated between being affectionate and hostile. At the present time, a separation action is pending, brought by the wife at the insistence of the Department of Public Welfare so that their aid to her may be legally correct. Nevertheless, they manage to see each other secretly and the enforced separation action is no indication of the real situation between them.

Mrs. A had extremely poor teeth with abscesses in her mouth. She had often been told that her teeth were a focus of infection. She complained of being fatigued all the time, was sick with frequent colds and had vaginal bleeding and abdominal pain after intercourse. In December, 1944, she had a perineal repair; a dilatation and curettage was performed in February, 1946.

The patient had no insight into the situation. Although she was constantly going to the agency for advice and help on every problem, she was not aware of the role she played in their marital problems. She felt that she was in a trap as far as her husband was concerned.

The husband had been a constant drinker and although he presented a pleasant appearance at times, he often talked like a wheedling child. His background indicated a good deal of nervous instability and he regarded himself as the black sheep of the family. He had served a prison term of four months for violation of parole, following his arrest in 1939 for the misappropriation of an automobile. In June, 1945, he was released after serving a three months term in the house of correction for assault and battery of his wife. He had been arrested on a number of occasions for drunkenness. He had been treated for alcoholism at a hospital where he gained weight and his tension decreased. At the hospital, it was considered that he had a borderline condition between a psychoneurosis and psychopathic personality. Comment was made upon his excessive dependence. Their child, whose father was the mother's first lover, was twelve years old, and undernourished, and had missed a great deal of school because of numerous colds and illnesses. She had been placed on at least four different occasions in different homes for a period of seven months. She had expressed the feeling that her mother did not love her, had inferiority feelings, was self-conscious and felt that people talked about her. In October, 1945, she was in a Society for the Prevention of Cruelty to Children temporary shelter for a few weeks and was referred to a Children's Clinic where she was seen once. One of the matrons commented that she was a love-starved child.

It might be of interest to apply to this family the five criteria of Rabbi Goldstein which we enumerated above:

(1) Legal: there had been numerous separations which did not lead to definite action on the initiative of either partner. In spite of constant difficulties and disagreements they were unable to reach a definite decision. The local Family Welfare Society had met as many financial needs as it could, but this proved to be insufficient and the D.P.W. had to implement considerably. In order to legal-ize their aid, the D.P.W. insisted that the wife prefer charges consistent with a separation action. The family had also had contact with the S.P.C.C. in reference to the daughter.

(2) Economic: the husband never contributed any money to the support of the family. The F.W.S. had already contributed sums for the hospital treatment of the husband and for recreational activities such as camp for the daughter.

(3) Biological: the mother complained constantly of fatigue and had abscessed teeth which were considered a focus of infection. She also had a gynecological disorder. The daughter has been sick with numerous illnesses and the husband was an alcoholic.

(4) Psychological: Mrs. A's behavior was unstable and erratic. Her father, who drank and deserted the family, was irresponsible. It is of significance that the patterns of be-havior in her husband resembled those of her own father in his drinking and in his irresponsibility. She had entertained rescue fantasies toward both of these men, her father and her husband, with the purpose of saving them from them-

selves. Her neurotic wish to be reunited with her father, was repeated in the numerous affairs which she had with men who were married or attached to another woman. She carried over a similar ambivalent attitude which she had toward her own unstable sister, to her daughter; in fact the daughter was named after this sister. The chief individuals involved, the patient, her husband, and her sister were sexually promiscuous and undependable. In the consideration of the entire problem there was concern as to what effects this atmosphere of instability, discord and disharmony would have upon the daughter who was just entering her adolescence.

(5) Ethical: ethical considerations are closely related to what has just been discussed under the psychological factors. The nature of the difficulties of the individuals concerned might be considered to be character neuroses, with manifestations in the characterological sphere. Thus, one is not surprised to find considerable moral laxness with its accompanying dissolution of family unity.

Although these five criteria have been considered separately for the purposes of the discussion, they are interrelated and interdependent. For example, from the legal aspect, the external pressure from the D.P.W. for separation action may have boomeranged in the opposite direction, so that the wife and husband secretly sought each other. In the economic sphere, the husband's inability to support the family aroused much resentment and hostility in the wife. Their conflicts in the psychological sphere accentuated and probably contributed considerably to the ill health of Mrs. A, especially in regard to her constant fatigue. In spite of the difficult reality factors, the emotional problems of the wife and husband were the most serious obstacles in the treatment by the social worker. The agency was informed that the wife had little to offer in constructive ways, that whatever help was given should be directed towards salvaging the twelve-year-old daughter. Supportive measures should be utilized with the wife and husband.

The second case which came under my personal observation is presented from the psychoanalytic point of view. It is an example of a couple in whom the external reality factors were of little significance but in whom their internal personal difficulties were paramount. Mrs. B, a highly intelligent, extremely sensitive, energetic and aggressive individual, had felt frustrated in her desires to attain recognition in a professional sphere. She grew up in a Jewish family in which the sons were highly favored and idolized. All the efforts of the family were concentrated on giving the most opportunities, especially educational, to the male members of the family. She, herself, worked at the sacrifice of her own education to further the professional pursuits of her brothers. She believed that she was neglected, that she was left out of the family circle and was most envious of her siblings who won the love of their mother. There was an intense sibling rivalry with both her brothers and sister. The conception of a close family circle became *over-evaluated,* and had the meaning of being loved, accepted, and secure: she began to feel resentful because she felt that she was rejected and excluded from this inner family circle. There was much bickering, quarreling and strife as reactions to her not being regarded as an important member of the family, and she finally developed a crusading spirit as to the importance and significance of a close family relationship.

She married a soft-spoken, kindly, business man, who was never ruffled by circumstances and who devoted his life to her welfare. In her fear of losing him, which, in her estimation, would result in disruption of her own family life, she became hostile towards the relatives of her husband, always fearing that they would try to take him away from her. Through the years of conflict with her husband in regard to her in-laws, the husband developed neurotic reactions to those individuals whom she felt threatened their family circle. He gave up all contacts with his own immediate family in order to maintain peace and to satisfy the possessiveness of his wife.

The domineering tendencies of Mrs. B were accepted by her husband whose needs to suffer and to be submissive were satisfied. The husband's mother had been a domineering possessive woman although more kindly disposed than Mrs. B. The more Mrs. B's husband yielded to her demands, which were manifested in intricate subtle ways, the greater was her own dissatisfaction with him. It so happened that she had hypochondriacal trends as a result of repressed hostile feelings. The husband, too, had had mild hypochondriacal trends, but in the later years of their marriage these became greatly accentuated, almost a *folie à deux*.

They had an only daughter and much effort was expended to create a close family spirit and maintain family solidarity.

Mrs. B was most jealous of any attention given to her daughter by her own siblings, always fearing that her daughter might be snatched away from her and be won over by them. At the same time she used the affection of her siblings for her daughter, as a means of trying to buy her way back into the good graces and love of her own family. The conflicts became so intense, that the only way to avoid strife was for this daughter to break off all contacts with her mother's relatives. When her daughter married, the same fears which Mrs. B had in regard to the relatives of her husband returned and expressed themselves concerning the relatives of the son-in-law. The neurotic need to preserve the intactness of her own family created an intolerable situation.

The in-laws of the daughter were forced to terminate their relationship to Mrs. B, just as her own relatives and the relatives of her husband had broken off contact with her. This, in turn, created conflicts between her daughter and her son-in-law and between the son-in-law and the mother. The tensions and problems increased to such a degree that it was necessary for the daughter to seek psychiatric help.

Mrs. B presented other psychiatric difficulties, but the main neurotic pattern which we wish to emphasize at this time, is the repetition of her neurotic need to restore the original intimate family circle in which she would be accepted by her family as the most loved child. One can readily understand how the daughter of this woman would unconsciously continue the fight of the mother to preserve the over-evaluated conception of the family circle on the basis of this infantile conflict. Thus the problems of the mother were repeated within the daughter and would be visited upon the next generation.

In spite of these negative factors which would seem sufficient to disrupt any marriage, superficially, the family appeared to outsiders a happy one, — a talented wife, a devoted husband and a loving daughter. Each partner possessed a strict conscience with high ethical standards which forced them to remain loyal to each other in spite of the neurotic needs to torture each other and to endure suffering.

In trying to understand marital problems, one must be aware of the combination of reality factors and the neurotic reactions of the partners. Usually, and especially in clients who seek aid from social service agencies, there is a combination of reality factors, chiefly in the economic sphere, and emotional difficulties as in the case of Mrs. A. In the patients whom one treats in private practice, the reality factors may be minimum with the preponderant weight in the direction of personal difficulties as in the case of Mrs. B. In general, one finds a complementary series in the combination of reality factors and neurotic reactions. If reality problems are extreme, the happiest of marriages in even so-called normal people may become disturbed. One may draw the analogy to neurotic soldiers with "battle fatigue," in which the external reality can be so severe and traumatic that the most normal of soldiers would succumb to neurotic behavior as a result of the severe current stress. Perhaps the reference to battle fatigue was suggested by the fact that marital is sometimes misspelled as martial — as a slip in writing.

Let us discuss those factors which contribute to the production of neurotic reactions. In general, it might be said that neurotics seek and find each other, the neurosis in one individual finds its counterpart in another: it is as if there were a phonograph record which is on the alert for a phonograph on which the neurotic plays his only tune. Edmund Bergler has aptly referred to these tendencies as "the unconscious synchronization of neurotic behavior patterns." In the case of Mrs. A, the client had the fantasy of rescuing her husband, who was in turn seeking someone to save him. In the case of Mrs. B her domineering, possessive and aggressive characteristics were fully accepted by her husband who was passive and had a need to suffer.

Some of the more specific factors in the production of neurotic reactions are:

(1) *The relative age of the partners:* if both partners are very young, the advantages of flexibility and plasticity for future adjustment to each other are present. On the other hand, the degree of immaturity may be so great, that there may be difficulty in assuming adult responsibilities and adjusting to reality. The problem of the young person who remains eternally adolescent can lead to difficulties

in that he brings to the situation attitudes and ideals that are anachronistic. The adolescent may still possess many illusions, idealizations, and expectations, far beyond what can actually be realized. This in turn leads to conflict, disappointment, and depression. If both partners are relatively old, for example in their late thirties, the aspect of a childless marriage is present and this may have unfavorable repercussions. If one of the partners is too young and the other too old, the usual pattern is a rather flagrant repetition of the old child-parent relationship; thus one of the partners will always remain as a child in the eyes of the other. Each, however, may be satisfying their inner longings of finding a parent who will love and protect him or her.

(2) *The perpetuation of unresolved infantile conflicts:* the passive man finds the aggressive woman and the struggle of submission and dominance can be played out and gratification of the unconscious need to suffer is attained. When the husband is insecure as to his abilities in the field of work and sex, he may seek to detach himself emotionally from his wife in an effort to become self-sufficient. Such behavior creates conflict in the type of woman who has excessive demands for love and protection, which in turn arouses the man's fears. In an effort to overcome the insistent demands of the wife, he becomes more detached, and the wife feels that this withdrawal on the man's part is an indication of her being rejected and she feels humiliated.

The advent of children, in addition to increasing the realistic factors of responsibility, may reactivate the old sibling rivalry situation giving rise to jealousy.

The savior complex, in which there is the effort to save the fallen man through marriage, *marriage of ambition,* in which feelings of inferiority are compensated for by the attainment of social status or the acquisition of money via the partner, become marriages of convenience with the elements of love playing little if any role. In *marriages of spite*, in which the son or daughter rebels and in revolt against the parental ideals marries someone out of their social class or some one of a different religion, the motive of revenge is quite strong.

(3) *Psychosexual problems* characterized by marital infidelity, jealousy, lack of affection and tenderness: the latter is especially poignant where sexual intimacy is considered as a purely physical satisfaction unaccompanied by warmth and tenderness.

The marital adjustment for the woman is more complicated and therefore more difficult than for the man. From the physiological standpoint, the psychosexual development as related to the menses, the period of child bearing and the menopause bring their own specific problems. In our present civilization in which there has been considerable emancipation of the woman, there is greater freedom in the expression of whatever masculine trends she may have. In war, masculine trends in women are especially accentuated; for example, their working in factories, their adoption of male attire and the assuming of greater responsibilities in the home. The return to homemaking and the giving up of wartime jobs suddenly puts a damper on such expression and the masculine trends must find other devious methods of satisfaction.

Unfortunately, at times marriage is recommended as a cure-all, almost like a patent medicine. Everybody likes to be considered normal and so to get into the swing of marriage provides proof of normalcy. To overcome feelings of loneliness and feelings of inferiority and inadequacy, marriage may be tried. It may be recommended as a solution for psychosexual difficulties and even psychosomatic disturbances.

In dealing with the problems of human beings we inevitably focus our attention on the abnormal and the pathological. Thus, although we have discussed certain aspects of marital problems, it is obvious that there are also positive factors which are conducive to happy and successful marriages. Perhaps there will come a time when we will be more interested in studying so-called normal people to determine what the forces are which maintain healthy adaptations. I do not propose at this time to discuss those factors that produce good marriages. In general, broken homes and disrupted marriages occur most often in those individuals whose problems are more in the sphere of what is known as character neurosis. The classical phychiatric terminolgy refers to these individuals as psychopathic personalities. If personalities are heavily weighted with psychopathy, characterized by tendencies toward instability, irresponsibility, and impulsiveness which militate towards unstable loose relationships, their marriage can easily be rendered asunder. It is not fortuitous that among clients who attend social service agencies, this particular problem looms higher than in private practice. In contrast to the facility with which this type of marriage may be dissolved is the stubborn, clinging persistence of compulsive neurotics to remain together. If we ask ourselves why this is, we know that the ethical standards and a sense of character are much more prominent in the compulsive neurotics in whom feelings of guilt, conscience, and a sense of morality are highly developed. If these two conceptions are applied to the case illustrations presented today, it is clear that in the case of Mrs. A and her husband, the dominant trends were in the direction of psychopathic behavior and thus the marriage was tenuous and vulnerable. In contrast, in spite of the intense suffering and personality disorders as evidenced in Mrs. B and her husband, we observe their endeavor to cling together and maintain a family unity just because of their own individual compulsive traits with concomitant high ethical standards.

Now, I will tell you a top military secret. From the experiences of the war, we noted that psychopathic individuals created the greatest difficulties for the army. On the other hand, the incidence of compulsion neurosis among soldiers who developed neurotic reactions and required hospitalization was the lowest. This would mean that those traits which we recognize as belonging to the compulsive neurotic such as respect for law and order, an inner sense of ethics, responsibility and inner discipline, forced them to continue the battle in spite of all adversity. I hope you will not get the impression that I am advocating that successful marriages will only occur in compulsive neurotics. What I would like to stress is the fact that the presence of such traits, although at times seemingly abnormal, may have positive values in the maintenance of a happy family life.

Marital problems must be viewed as a facet of the family which is recognized as the cornerstone of our civilization. There is a close relationship among the family, the community and society. We know how important and significant the integrity of the family is for good personal adjustment. As our knowledge in social work and psychiatry has advanced, we have become much more careful and think twice before advising the placement of children in foster homes on the basis of what the deprivation of a mother means, and the traumatic effects of separation.

Marriage counseling should remain within the province of the social worker, minister, and with a psychiatrist on call to assist with personal problems as is the practice with any other personality problem in case work. There should be a close integration of case work, religion, psychiatry and the court. A model for such a relationship has been established in many courts for juvenile delinquency in which the psychiatrist presents his findings and recommendations. It would seem that such methods should be included for those individuals on the brink of divorce.

Couples who have marital difficulties would do well to seek advice first from their minister. If the problems are superficial and acute, the minister can deal with them at the level of counseling; if, however, a problem is chronic and of long standing, a deeper probing and psychiatric treatment may be necessary. The minister can prepare a couple by indicating the need for psychiatric help, orienting the couple as to what this means so that they will seek such treatment.

Well trained psychiatrists are very careful not to advise marriage or divorce. They believe that these are vital and significant decisions which must be left to the individual concerned. The attitude of the psychiatrist is perforce one of neutral sympathy. He tries to make clear to what extent the difficulties are neurotic and then to help the individual solve his problems through overcoming his neurosis. With the freedom from neurosis, the individual attains a sufficient degree of maturity so that he himself can make his own decisions.

NOTE: In gathering material for this lecture I am indebted to the following:

Bergler, E., "Synchronization of Neurotic Behavior Patterns." *Am. J. Med. Sci.*, 210, 470, Oct., 1945.

Bergler, E., *Unhappy Marriage and Divorce*. N. Y. Internat. Universities Press, 1946.

Goldstein, S. E., *Marriage and Family Counseling*. McGraw-Hill Book Co., Inc., N. Y., 1945.

Michaels, J. J., "Strength Through Character." *Am. J. Orthopsychiat.* 16: 350, April, 1946.

Michaels, J. J., and Porter, R. T., "The Striking Contrast in the Incidence of Compulsion Neurosis and Psychopathic Personality in the Armed Forces, Psychiatric and Social Implications." Accepted for Publication in *J. Nerv. and Ment. Dis.*

Mittleman, B., "Complementary Neurotic Reactions in Intimate Relationships." *Psychoanal. Quart.* 13: 479, 1944.

Discussion: ERIC F. MACKENZIE

Professor Magoun stated that one of the reasons why true love is so very rare and why the perfectly happy marriage doesn't eventuate quite as often as we wish it would, is something in the way of defective training — that people weren't properly prepared, and they don't change just because they go through a ceremony. People, selfish and so forth, remain selfish after the first thrill of romance is gone by. They had these traits before they entered into the marriage and they continue there to operate badly. That, of course, is perfectly sound psychology.

I'd like to submit one idea in reference to this matter of training. When the whole of public opinion, relatively speaking, is encouraging young folks to approach marriage with the idea that it's "something to do," "something which you try," but something which, if it doesn't work out well, can be discarded with a minimum of effort: it seems to me that there is a considerable premium being placed upon the development of a purely personal, purely selfish norm in regard to marriage, and upon it, therefore, the expectation in advance that whenever difficulties arise, that's a pretty good time to break the marriage up.

It is a matter of history that, a hundred years or so ago, people approached marriage with the idea that it was pretty permanent. There was, if you will, no escape. Now that could make for unhappiness in individual cases — seemingly tragic. In other cases, it had this benefit — it forced people to have a good deal more patience, a good deal more determined personal effort to make good than I observe to be present in many of these tragic cases which come my way today. Professor Magoun suggested just this idea, and I am simply amplifying what he said in that regard.

Marriage, like anything else, is something you have to

work for, something you have got to stay with, something you have to believe in. If you do all that, if you really believe in it, believe it is something you can give your best self to, and, therefore, give yourself to continuously, steadily, in spite of temporary difficulties — if we develop that idea, we will have more happy homes, we will have a better population, less juvenile delinquency and all the other consequences that go with broken homes.

We Catholics tell our people that marriage is permanent, that the institution of civil divorce, which is so common in our day, is not for them. I am not saying that our teaching is successful — it certainly isn't — but at least it is an ideal which we hold to. The mere fact that that ideal is not reached, in our mind, is not a reason for dropping the ideal itself. I was very happy to find indications of recognition of that from the point of view of psychologists and psychiatrists — that there is more real happiness in the idea of permanence, the idea of having a goal, an ideal which is so fine and so high that it can be worked for and worked for hard and steadily and permanently. This is something which commends itself to their scientific judgment.

In conclusion, it can be seen that there is a close relationship between the fields of religion and psychiatry especially concerning marriage. Rabbi Goldstein described five factors, (1) legal (2) economic (3) biological (4) psychological and (5) ethical, which are helpful in evaluating marital problems. An attempt was made to illustrate the application of these five criteria in the discussion of Mrs. A. From the psychiatric point of view, in which psychological difficulties were predominant, the case of Mrs. B. was presented. Usually there is a complementary series in the relative interaction of reality factors and neurotic reactions. Some of the general considerations which have psychologic significance are: the tendency of the neurotic partner to find his neurotic counterpart; the relative age of the partners, the perpetuation of unresolved infantile conflicts; psychosexual problems and the utilization of marriage as psychotherapy. Finally marital problems must be viewed as a facet of the family. There should be a close integration between the social worker, minister, psychiatrist and the court.

Discussion: HENRY H. WIESBAUER

One of the most important things about these two days of meeting is that they *are being held.* In how many other places can such a group as is gathered here, meet and attempt to pool the ideas of these several professions?

The two papers just presented, it seems to me, are good cases in point. All of us — clergymen, psychiatrists, medical men, social workers, nurses — from whatever profession we come, get the feeling of concern for individual people and for families and, most definitely, for the whole of the community. For the emphasis on individual families, as Dr. Liebman has shown, is carried to its logical conclusion in the whole community.

In Dr. Michaels' paper, I was impressed with the fact that he saw this given family in one of the cases in the social context. He points out the woman in her early thirties who looked liked forty. This was preceded by his mentioning that the family agencies need more adequate funds and how the family income had to be supplemented by the D.P.W.

We sensed the personal social dynamics (as he brought them to bear in his thinking and treatment of this family) and the realization for us, as professional people, that somehow what we are talking about in meetings like this — the knowledge that comes — must get out to the factories, to the labor union halls and the National Association of Manufacturers, the Chamber of Commerce; and we must come to bring this, regardless of cost and where the chips fall, to the knowledge of our families and our people.

He mentioned social sins and the need for modern prophets who will learn from psychiatry and allied fields what social forces work together to break up families and cause anxieties. This morning, you will find people who are wondering how they will pay for their dinner tonight as a part of family life. There is a need to get wise men all over our country to consider the human factor, and how a man's vocation and a woman's job makes each of them feel about marriage and their children.

Finally, in Dr. Michaels' paper, the sense of understanding of the need for professional teamwork, to me, was quite impressive. I noticed he seemed to feel that one of his most fortunate experiences in the service was his contact with other professional people. It seems to me that one of the things he was saying was that the Army and Navy provided situations for professional people to meet which peacetime does not provide. Think of it — when we kill, we get together; when we heal, we separate, and our people — those in trouble, those with marital problems, those with family problems, — cannot find us.

I was impressed that the Doctor and his staff went to Sunday services and also with the fact that, just so, the chaplains were invited to come to staff conferences. Here is, in my opinion, the professional spirit for which the world is crying out, and symposiums like this give me courage when I know that, as a clergyman, the professions are coming to recognize that religion has something to say, and I am trying to learn how to say it more clearly, in language that other professions can understand. I feel I have much to learn and have a great debt to psychiatry, to psychology, to medicine, to all these areas in our categorical thinking, through which, down the ages and today, I believe God Himself is trying to speak to us if we will listen and look beneath the language of a given profession to the content, to the meaning.

At the training level, in the universities, and in the professional schools — how much orientation have you as to other professions? For example, I am thinking now in this country — let's make it general — of one of the schools of social work where there are, in a nearly two-year program, three hours given to understanding religion — one on the Roman Catholic position, one on the Jewish position, and one on the Protestant position — and that is the orientation in the field of religion. At least that is more than some schools of social work are offering. Some offer nothing. And yet we send people forth in that profession to explore those things which are of importance to people's feelings and in their lives.

I wonder if, at the professional level, psychiatry is not challenging all of us to give more specific orientation to, for example, psychiatry to nursing, psychiatry to family case work, and to general medicine, so that, when a man or woman with a marital problem comes to our office, we can recognize in the first interview that this man has an ulcer, as well as the fact that he comes in saying "I had an argument with my wife, and I'm not going home."

One can read in the field of psychiatry very convincing and helpful and specific illustrations, but among the religious community, where can we find documentary evidence in individual cases and families, where the power and the understanding and dynamics of religion are illustrated, if you will, on a case basis? Too often, I think, we take recourse to a phrase I have heard often in meetings similar to this, that "religion is the plus."

I believe the church needs to define the "plus," just as the psychiatrist is putting up, as it were, what he does and what he has to offer and showing us the results in people's lives. And so I think that those of us in the religious community are receiving a legitimate challenge to consider as one of our approaches a clinical approach.

As a clergyman, I believe that intelligent religion (with a line under the word "intelligent") can supply that need. I believe that those of us who are in the strictly religious field are challenged by the clinical methods of psychiatry, to show in clinical terms what happens specifically when persons are religious in an intelligent sense.

In Professor Magoun's paper he said, "We dream about ends without much thought of means." And in the same section, "The word 'love' is not the thing 'love.'" It is my personal opinion that in the rank and file of the religious community we daydream very much about the ends, but are too specifically or intelligently concerned about the means. For instance, in the field of marital counseling, not long ago, there came to my office a married woman. As she talked, for perhaps an hour, one could clearly see the need for psychiatric attention. Yet, a well-known member of her denomination had recommended to her that she take up bicycle riding as the solution to her difficulties — a woman fifty years of age who weighs over two hundred pounds!

I believe our danger as clergymen, as we take more and more interest in the field of psychiatry and allied sciences, is that we will tend to take our functional concepts from professions which are not legitimately ours. Let me illustrate.

Recently, there came to my office a man of about fifty years of age. He appeared to be a person who was on the verge of giving up. That is, his beard, while not fully grown, had been neglected for two or three days; his clothing, while not completely untidy, was in the process of becoming untidy. And both in his attitude and in his appearance, one saw the possibility that, without some hope, he *would* give up and, in another week, would reach that classification some people call a "bum." He wanted

money from me. If there is one thing our culture understands, it's that, and I felt his concern. His asking that of
us, as a religious group, was a legitimate thing. He wanted
it for something to eat and a bed for the night. We co-
operate with one of the social settlement houses, and I
arranged this on the telephone. The man got up to go, and
I asked him to sit down a moment if he was not in a hurry.
I asked him if he was married. "My wife died six years
ago," he told me, in broken English. "I go to mental hospital; I can't live without her. I sick. I stay there six months
and better; I come out." I said, "Are there children in your
family?" By then in tears, he said, "Two boys. One boy
killed in accident next year after wife died; other boy die in
football game, one year later. I all alone. All alone; nobody
care."

A few nights later, at a meeting of professional people,
I sat next to a clergyman who had been taking special
training in the field of psychiatry and religion. We fell to
talking about persons who come to the religious community
with financial needs as a part of their problem, and he began to describe this man. I discovered that his institution
had turned away the man for whom I found food and a
place to sleep — had, in fact, turned him away the same day,
before he came to the Pastoral Counseling Center. This
young professional man said, "We brushed him off. From
our point of view, he doesn't have any growth potential."

Here religion does have a part to play in helping all
of us in the professions, who work with families in trouble.
We are all children of God; let us remember that a man's
creed and his color and his social status and cultural background and his "growth potential" are all secondary to the
fact that he is a child of God and is entitled to our help.

Finally, as we see the individual, as we see family life,
we think in religious groups of that larger family to which
our chairman referred, God's family — the religious com-

munity. Here, in times of personal stress, at best, the religious community can provide a larger group amongst whom there is warmth and understanding and love and acceptance and concrete help.

CHAPTER TEN

THE GRIEF SITUATION
Henry H. Brewster

GRIEF IS ORDINARILY CONSIDERED to be a normal reaction of a person to a distressing situation. But psychiatrists, especially Dr. Erich Lindemann,[1] (with whom I am associated at Harvard University), have been interested in grief as it represents a specific reaction to a traumatic human experience.

Our contact with grief has been only in terms of patients whom we have seen at the hospital. In particular, it has concerned relatives of victims both of the Cocoanut Grove fire and of fatal disease, as well as psychoneurotics who have lost a relative after their hospital admission. One can see, therefore, that our experience with grief is limited to a few compared to the many who are seen outside a hospital by the clergyman.

As we have observed it, acute grief is a definite reaction with physical and psychological manifestations. It occurs immediately after a distressing situation or after a period of delay. There may be complete absence of grief, or there may be a distorted picture of grief. We have, as a result, separated grief into what we call a normal and a morbid reaction. From a normal grief reaction a person may recover without psychiatric help. A patient will not recover from a morbid grief reaction without the help of an expert.

But first, the normal grief reaction. The picture is fairly uniform. We have a person who complains of great somatic distress coming in waves which last ten to twenty minutes.

---

[1] Lindemann, E., "Symptomatology and Management of Acute Grief," *American Journal of Psychiatry*, 101: 141-148, 1944.

There is a need to sigh. There is a hollow feeling in the stomach, a dry feeling in the throat, choking and difficulty in breathing, and a distressing subjective sensation which the patient describes as tension or mental pain.

Particularly conspicuous seems to be the sigh respiration. Another striking symptom is the loss of muscular power. The bereaved has different ways of speaking of it. He finds it a great effort to walk to the street corner; his arms will feel heavy; it is all he can do to climb a flight of stairs. A common bodily symptom is related to the stomach. The patient will say that food tastes like sand; he "stuffs" it into himself. It is apparent that the bereaved person is extremely anxious to avoid the discomfort that he is suffering. This discomfort can be accentuated by mentioning the deceased, by the visits of friends, or by the expression of sympathy: the bereaved will avoid, with the greatest effort, being reminded of the deceased.

There is a definite change in the mental status of the patient. He will complain of a feeling of unreality; he recognizes an emotional distance from other people: they seem small or shadowy.

Finally, there is an inescapable preoccupation with the image of the deceased. This is a dramatic symptom. A Navy pilot lost a pal during the war, and he found that after the pal had died, he had an imaginary companion. His pal was with him at all his meals; he would talk to him, and they would discuss plans for the future. The pilot found this a very distressing symptom and he had the feeling that he was going insane.

Another serious preoccupation is that of guilt. The bereaved searches his past life to find any way that he has failed to do right by the person that died. He exaggerates minor omissions, and he berates himself for not having treated the deceased better. A man lost his wife in the Cocoanut Grove fire. The situation was that he and his wife were leaving Cocoanut Grove at the same time. He fainted and somebody dragged his body out, but his wife was burned to death. He felt that he was responsible for not having saved his wife.

Another reaction of which a patient complains is lack of emotional warmth. He finds that he is responding to situations with anger and irritability; people bother him. And this happens at a most unfortunate moment, because it is at that time that relatives and friends are attempting to maintain a friendly atmosphere. This show of hostility is perplexing to a patient: he cannot account for it, and he feels, again, that he is going insane.

The first grief patient that I treated was referred to me by the pediatric department because she had been abusive to her twelve-year-old son. It became apparent that she was quite emotionally disturbed — very prone to cry. Soon, her only topic of conversation was her husband who had died in the hospital following an operation. She painted an ideal picture of him, as if he were the best-looking man in the world, as if he had treated her better than any husband could, as if she had received from him everything she wanted in terms of money and of opportunity. As we reviewed together the memories of her husband, we found that actually her true predominating feeling was that of hostility towards him. It turned out, in fact, that he had been quite incompetent, very rarely at home, had never given her any opportunities, but that she had felt unable to leave him. So we see that the hostile feelings towards her husband had been so painful for this woman that she had transferred them by the process of displacement to her son, where they became more tolerable for her.

A final characteristic of the acute grief reaction is what we choose to call a loss of former patterns of conduct. We find that a person experiencing grief is not necessarily retarded in his thought and in his actions — in fact, his talk may show a push and he may be exceedingly restless, moving about in an aimless way unable to find what he wants. He seems unable to initiate and maintain useful patterns of conduct — instead, he moves around with no purpose, and the things that he does seem to fall apart into pieces as if each piece were a great task. He becomes aware of the fact that his usual behavior has been extremely dependent upon a meaningful relationship with the deceased. This means that the patient becomes quite dependent upon a person who can provide him with comfort, and who can help to initiate actions for him. This is not true only of grief of course. It can also be said of a person who is depressed.

We can now say that acute grief, as we have seen it, is the reaction of an individual when he or she ceases to interact with a meaningful person, lost by death or separation. The tell-tale signs of this reaction will be bodily symptoms of distress and loneliness, preoccupation with the image of the deceased, guilt, hostility reactions, and a loss of the normal patterns of useful conduct.

About the course of normal grief. It appears to be a condition which can be helped materially within eight or ten interviews, and from which one should recover within three to four weeks. There are obstacles in the way of this recovery. I have already indicated that a person experiencing grief will make every effort to avoid the distressing feelings. Therefore, the duration of grief will depend upon the capacity of the person to face the bereavement situation, to tolerate the feeling of distress, to relive the memory of the deceased person.

Now I would like to say a word about the morbid grief reaction, and I am going to skip over it because it does lead us, I think, a little afield. But, just to mention characteristics of morbid grief reaction:

The most common thing that happens is delay in the grief process — delay or even postponement. We know that this delay can last as long as twenty years. We have had the experience of seeing a woman of forty who lost her husband. She had what appeared to be an excessive grief reaction: she was totally and completely incapacitated. But the degree of her grief could not be accounted for by the severity of her loss. As it turned out in therapy, her emotion was more concerned with a brother who had died twenty years previously. We now know that when two grief reactions like this occur together the response, the grief, can be extremely severe.

Then there are various distortions of the picture of grief. There may be great overactivity on the part of a person without a sense of loss; instead, the patient is full of zest and tends to engage in adventuresome and expansive projects. We know of a man, aged fifty, who had lost his wife and was beginning to recover from his state of grief. He suddenly was filled with the urge to sell all his furniture, his house, and everything that had to do with the memory of his wife. He was persuaded not to do this on the basis that he was running away from his grief.

Another indication of morbid grief reaction is that of medical disease itself. We have found that in cases of ulcerative colitis and rheumatoid arthritis, there are definite relationships to a grief situation.

I have spoken of the hostility with which the bereaved responds to persons round about him. There may be furious hostility directed against an individual, as against the doctor who operated upon the deceased. Or we may see a wooden sort of a person who moves around like a robot and shows no emotional activity whatsoever. The most serious complications of grief are found in a person who loses permanently his patterns of useful, social interaction, or who develops an agitated depression with suicidal tendencies.

A brief word on the prognosis of grief. There seems to

ationship between the severity of grief and
nteraction which formerly existed between
the deceased. This interaction, this re-
of the bereaved to the deceased, need not have
been affectionate—it may have been a hostile one, in which
the bereaved did not have opportunity to express this hostility because of social status or of relationship or of some
other factor. We find that mothers who lose young children
have a particularly severe reaction. People of obsessive
personalities who have been subject to previous depressions
are likely to have very severe grief.

The management of grief is not the sole province of the
psychiatrist. We know, of course, that the church has handled the problem of grief for a long time and with great
effectiveness. There are certainly thousands of people who
are experiencing grief and do not need to make their way
to any special person outside of their family.

In terms of what I have said about the acute grief reaction, we can note and interpret certain phenomena often
taking place in the progress of grief. We know, after a
person dies, that the bereaved is visited by friends; flowers
of great beauty are sent to the house; the priest, or minister,
or rabbi, may call: much is done to diminish the tension
and discomfort of the bereaved. At the church service, at
the funeral, a group of friends and relatives are together
and the bereaved is brought into interaction with other
people again; there is an exchange of remarks about the
deceased, especially concerning what a wonderful person
he was. If an obituary is delivered, it tends to idealize the
deceased. In the mourning period that follows the funeral,
the bereaved may make a great effort to recall the image
of the deceased. Then, perhaps, we come to a period of
pastoral counseling. Here the dogma of the church, depending on the individual's belief, may come to his relief.
Where the bereaved believes that he has been villainous

toward and neglectful of the deceased, his religious belief may indicate that it was not his villainy but the will of God that caused the death of the deceased. Finally, the bereaved may have hope of the life hereafter in which he will meet the deceased and make up for the things that he didn't do right. Such a belief would be helpful in reducing the guilt of the bereaved. We can classify these phenomena as means of rendering comfort to the bereaved.

Providing comfort alone, however, does not resolve the grief reaction. In the people we have seen at the hospital, depression follows this period of comforting. It is necessary, after this period of comforting, for the bereaved to find a sympathetic person, be he psychiatrist, minister, or friend, who gives him a feeling of understanding and assists him in reviewing the emotional experiences he has shared with the deceased. The tendency of the bereaved person is to idealize the deceased. He may even have been thinking of the deceased as an imaginary figure. With the help of the therapist, it is necessary for the bereaved to consider the deceased as a real person, as a real loss, before he can readjust to, and make new relations in, a world in which the deceased is missing.

I have perhaps given the impression to you that it is easy to take hold of a bereaved person and to assist him. This is not always so. Sometimes he will reject our efforts to help him. Then it is necessary to find support in the family or a social worker or a friend who will bring the bereaved person to us until he can tolerate the discomfort of grieving.

A reaction similar to the grief state can occur without a person dying. It may follow a period in which there has been a separation of two people, as in the case of a war when one partner of a marriage goes into the armed services. Then we run into a paradoxical situation in which a grief reaction occurs but is inappropriate. That is what Dr.

Lindemann has called an anticipatory grief reaction. I would like to give an example because it does seem to be relevant to certain veteran problems that have confronted us.

A wife loses her husband in the war. I say "loses," implying that the husband has gone overseas. All sorts of thoughts have occurred to her about how he may die. She adjusts herself to a life in which he is missing. She has, at last, almost reached the point of living in a world in which he does not exist. She is not interested in other men. Then, he returns from the Army. He finds her completely cold: she is in a state of grief reaction over her "loss" of him, and our job is to unwind this reaction.

In summary, grief work consists in the emancipation of the bereaved from the bondage of the deceased. Then the bereaved can readjust himself to a world in which the deceased is missing. Finally he will find new human relationships which fill the place of those lost by the death of the deceased.

Discussion: SUZANNE TAETS VAN AMERONGEN

Dr. Brewster has made a distinction between normal grief reactions and morbid grief reactions. I should like, in the first place, to elaborate on grief reactions as we see them in children.

Here in America, I have worked with children, and have seen many children who come from families where father or mother suddenly died, and have dealt with their special problems. There is a feeling, sometimes, that death and the problems of life and death should be kept from the child. Even if there is a loss in the family — father goes into the Army and one day there is a message that he will not come back and has died overseas — mother is often very embarrassed: how shall she explain to the child what happened? She had thought that it was not necessary to prepare a child for the problems of death, and that those problems are, more or less, beyond the child's understanding.

What happens when a child loses one of his family, and especially when a mother dies? We can see the same symptoms that Dr. Brewster has mentioned; we see them in the child, too. Of course, they are a little bit more simplified. For the child, death is something which he cannot understand, and it is very difficult to compete with the idea that "mother just never will come back."

We see that in children the hostility factor is of very much more importance — the child often interprets the death of father or mother as a "being left" and the hostile reactions are much less covered up than they are in adults.

The same thing happens when the mother in the family is bereaved and has to go through the grief process Dr. Brewster pictured for you. Very often, the child, at that time, more or less lacks attention from the mother — the mother is too busy with herself, trying to settle her problems — and there often is the tendency to assume that one can better take the child away and not discuss any more what happened at home because the child will not understand and the child is dragged away as soon as the ceremonies for burial and so on take place. We, later on, very often get those children at the clinic with very outspoken hostile reactions, not at all unaware of what's been going on, but with very definite notions.

It seems to me important for ministers and rabbis to realize the fact, as they come into families where some catastrophe has taken place, that even a child of two or three has a subtle consciousness of what's going on, and you cannot just go about it by dragging him away and not discussing the event any further.

Especially with children, there is a curiosity connected with the problems of death and life, and a child will be apt to ask all sorts of details — "What happened to mother when she got put in the coffin and they put her under the earth?" and "What will happen to her now?" and "How did she get to Heaven?" All those very concrete and practical questions a child must ask, and an adult will have to answer them, enabling the child to adjust to death, and giving him the opportunity to accept death as something which belongs in his life as it belongs in all our lives.

There is one other thing I should like to point out with respect to morbid grief reactions. I come from a country where we have suffered from deportation; and, especially, there are people who went through very bad experiences in imprisonment and in concentration camps. We expected that when those people came back, they would immediately show more or less neurotic symptoms and collapse. Many of us were astonished to see that those people had been able to go through terrible experiences. They therefore already presented a certain selection in physical and moral strength. At first they seemed to be rather well adjusted, they were a little bit more quiet, a little bit more withdrawn. One had the feeling that contact wasn't quite as it had been before, but things seemed to move along rather well. The families were very happy, and soon were so used to having this person back, that they took him for granted. After a few weeks, the feeling that "now things were as they were before," came, especially with regard to the women who had to resume their household duties, their responsibilities; the men who were in good health were allowed to relax for a while, but then everybody talked about new opportunities and new jobs and things like that.

I know two cases from personal experience: a man who came back — one of forty out of 1500 who returned — and one of a woman who came back from one of the women's concentration camps in Berlin, and seemed to adjust rather well, but, after a few months, collapsed in indefinite physical complaints. At first, we thought her complaint was more like nervous pain — neuralgia. After that, she didn't seem to react to the usual medication that we give neuralgia patients, and we then saw that she had dropped into a state of total apathy, of disinterest in surroundings, and total lack of responsibility — as someone reported it once to me, a feeling that "well, the world is just going on, but there is no meaning left."

As you deal with people who come from European countries, and especially as the problem of displaced persons becomes more acute, I should not be surprised if you would, in one way or another, deal with some of these, "delayed reactions," even though there is not always the problem of having an actual death or bereavement situation.

Discussion: DR. LIEBMAN

I learned in my work with Dr. Lindemann right after the Cocoanut Grove disaster that the grief situation is, indeed, a very complex one. It is often difficult to distinguish appearance from reality. Sometimes when death comes other members of the family are made to pay a terrible price because of the loss of one member of the family circle.

I had an experience in the midwest a number of years ago which remains vivid in my memory. A certain professional man lost a very brilliant son and all the rest of his children suffered terribly from the father's rejection. Undoubtedly he did reject them, making them feel that they were as nothing compared with the son that was lost. Of course again and again he protested to me how much he loved his children, but as I look back upon the situation now, I realize that he was making them pay a great price for being alive.

Often when grief comes we torment ourselves with guilt

feelings that quite frequently are unjustified. A letter came to me this past year from a very brilliant and charming woman in her seventies who, a few weeks before writing me, had lost her beloved helpmate after forty years of joyous marriage. After his death she tormented herself by thinking of the things that she had done or not done. I wrote her pointing out that undoubtedly she had been a marvelous wife to her husband; I could sense the devotion in every line that she had written. She told me that she had read the chapter on grief in "Peace of Mind" (which is, of course, the fruit of the work with Dr. Lindemann) and that it had come as a kind of revelation to her — that guilt feelings are natural and universal and that we can expect no detour around grief. It takes even the strongest and most normal persons weeks or months to readjust to a genuine loss.

Another letter came to me recently from a woman in the South who expressed gratitude for Dr. Lindemann's healing insight, that we must not be afraid to express our sorrow when we genuinely feel it, and that harsh repression of the emotion of grief is indeed a dangerous procedure. After she had lost a dear one, her minister told her, "You must be brave — be a stoic — control your emotions." As the months passed she began to be afflicted with a number of psychosomatic symptoms as a result of this ruthless repression of her feelings. She was helped greatly when a wise physician applying the techniques of Dr. Lindemann enabled her to work through her bereavement burden.

General Discussion

QUESTION: Isn't lack of sleep one of the severe symptoms of grief? How would you handle that?

DR. BREWSTER: I should have mentioned sleeplessness

when I was talking about the loss of former patterns of social conduct, of restlessness, of the inability to sit still, and of the pressure to keep on the move without knowing where one is moving. It certainly is a prominent characteristic and demands the use of sedation.

QUESTION: It has been my experience that the concepts of immortality and Heaven, which the first speaker mentioned, have, to a large extent, lost their reality for people today. If so, how can we, as clergymen, utilize those things as sources for help in the grief situation?

DR. BREWSTER: The concepts of immortality and Heaven cannot be utilized to afford comfort to the bereaved if they are foreign to his religious beliefs.

QUESTION: Dr. Brewster stated in his paper that it was a teaching of the church that the death of the deceased was the will of God. I wonder if that belief is prevalent among psychiatrists.

DR. BREWSTER: I mentioned the will of God not as a teaching of the church or as the belief of psychiatrists, but as a possible belief of the bereaved. If the bereaved did not believe in this concept, it would be of no use in the treatment of his grief reaction.

QUESTION: What about small children (say, from two years of age up to ten) attending funerals? Do you regard this as wise or unwise from the psychiatric point of view?

DR. VAN AMERONGEN: I think the problem is not so much whether we should have children attend certain social, or certain religious ceremonies that I would say belong to the adult life and do not, in the same way, belong to the child's life. I don't think that it is necessary, and I don't even think that one should wish that small children attend all those ceremonies. On the contrary, I should say that we have seen very often that a child who attended those ceremonies at an age when he was not able to understand them, to integrate them, is done more harm than good.

But I think that very often the parents or other people are apt to say, "Well, the whole problem of death is beyond the child," and I don't think that that is true. From experience, we know that the child, even before it can talk, as soon as it visualizes its ideas even in dreams, has certain ideas about death. Sleep and death, for a child, are often alike. For instance, after death has happened in a family, the child is afraid to go to sleep because it has the idea that one just lies down and doesn't know whether he will get up.

I think it is always a necessity to verbalize in terms that the child can understand. Before this psychiatric era, there existed the conception that death and sex were topics that a child couldn't understand. Actually, it was the parent that didn't know how to tell about it. I think that is the major problem; I don't think it is the major problem that the child can't understand, because a child can understand very well if one knows how to talk in terms of the child and if one has the patience to give the child the opportunity to talk about it and to ask questions. What very often happens is that one says, "Well, I don't know — grandfather went away," or "Father just left," which is much worse than giving to the child a certain explanation and a certain verbalizing that something very difficult to accept and sad has happened.

I think that this doesn't mean that, therefore, the child has to attend the ceremonies, which is something different.

DR. LIEBMAN: I would like to add a word from experiences

that I have had in the last several years. I think that children should not be excluded from family sorrow. I feel more and more that children are very sensitive about being put into exile and, if exiled from the family circle, no matter what rationalization may be given, they feel it.

In my pastoral work I discovered this truth in an unforgettable way. I officiated at the funeral of the father of a good friend of mine. After the services, the parents told me that they had sent their seven-year-old son away as soon as they had learned of the father's death. "You see, we wanted to shield our boy from the sorrow here in the household . . . so we sent him to the home of a cousin of ours in a neighboring suburb." I asked whether the boy had ever been away from home and what his feelings were toward these strange cousins. When I learned that this was his first expulsion from the family circle, that he was exiled without any real explanation, I told the father and mother that they were trying to shield him from participating in their own emotional life and were imposing upon him a much greater psychic strain through separation from his loved ones and a general feeling of uncertainty and mystery. "What shall we do, then?" asked the parents. "Bring him back home," I said. "Tell him what I am sure he already knows, that his grandfather has died and that he is needed to cheer up his Daddy. The parents followed my advice and found that their seven-year-old son was quite aware of what had happened, although he was afraid to talk of the death of his grandfather, and that he was, indeed, beginning to feel an "outsider" until he was given a role to play in the circle of family life.

Children understand much more than we usually realize. They can take truth, but they cannot easily take deception or what seems to them to be deception. Children, when it becomes necessary, can stand sorrow much better than exclusion, lies or pretense from the very people they trust most, their father and mother.

QUESTION: What will you tell a child of, say, four to six years of age, concerning death?

DR. LIEBMAN: When I have been faced with this question from parents, "Shall we tell our child grandfather is gone to Heaven?" I acquiesce, if this is the formula and pattern which is experienced in the family. In other words, I do not believe that a child, four to six, should be subjected to abstract theological argumentation.

I know that there are a great many profound questions that perturb children — the fear of rejection, the fear of the dark, of aloneness, the fears of anger and hostility. Many of these fears are associated with death in the child's mind.

Paul Schilder, a very great authority in this field, in *The Goals and Desires of Man*, published by the Columbia University Press, a very technical work in psychoanalysis, has a whole chapter dealing with the thoughts and fears of death on the part of children as well as adults.

Now ofttimes we make the mistake of dealing with problems that are not cogent or not real. Actually most children want to feel a sense of warm security at the time of death, of warm belongingness to the circle of sorrow. If they are given this feeling, they will not ask theological or metaphysical questions as frequently as will the rejected child or the child who is left with mystery. The boy or girl who is excluded or exiled will have terrified thoughts about death, resulting in abstract theological questions.

I think, in other words, that the child should be dealt with on his own level, and should be given simple answers and also an extra dosage of love at that particular time, an extra dosage of security and belongingness to a circle that protects. That is the way I handle the problem when it confronts me as a rabbi.

QUESTION: How do you explain the desire of some families to have the bodies of soldiers killed in service returned to them from cemeteries overseas?

DR. BREWSTER: If the family chooses to have a coffin returned from overseas, we can assume from what we have learned in our work that there is a remnant of the grief state remaining. While the body of the deceased is overseas, the family may have an *idealized* memory of the deceased. When the body is at home, the family may find it easier to deal with the *actual* image of the deceased and to complete their grief reaction.

The same could be said about open coffins at funerals. If it is of assistance for the individual to complete grief work, then it is a legitimate measure.

QUESTION: I should be interested to have a comparison between the grief situations of men and women: first, as to the comparative number of men and women who seek expert help in such situations; and, second, as to the difference, if any, in the reaction under these similar situations, of men and women.

DR. BREWSTER: I think that we can take as an example in answering this question, a situation that prevailed after the Cocoanut Grove fire, where there was a fair representation of both men and women undergoing the grief reaction.

The men experiencing grief were, in general, very tense and resistant to being interviewed. Dr. Lindemann cites a man who was exceedingly hostile to him when interviewed within the hospital. In fact, this man remained inaccessible for psychotherapy.

It is possible, however, to sell the idea to a man. It may possibly be more difficult for him to give in to tears and the feeling of discomfort. We have had no good clinical evidence to indicate that a grief reaction is qualitatively different between sexes.

QUESTION: What clinical showing is there of sex frustation in women, after bereavement, as contributing to psychosomatic disturbances?

DR. BREWSTER: I should say that sexual frustration can occur in the male as well as in the female as a result of the grief situation. An example will, perhaps, put the point more clearly.

A woman lost her husband during the war. When she received word of his death, she did feel dejected for a period of time, but not very much so. During the ensuing two years, she became very active in the management of her husband's business. Friends noticed that she was always on the go, but outwardly calm. Several eligible men wanted to marry her. But she could not accept marriage, despite the pressing need of her children to have a father. The reason she could not marry became apparent later.

At the time she learned of her husband's death, her youngest daughter developed nightmares in which she believed there was a man in the house. "The man" was of course her dead father about whom mother talked so incessantly, to whom mother gave so much love which her daughter should have received. Mother had, in fact, failed to emancipate herself from the idealized image of her dead husband. No wonder she could not marry again and provide her daughter with a real father.

QUESTION: About a month after the bereavement, the clergyman calls on the bereaved. Is it wise for the clergyman to wait until the bereaved person alludes to the one who has gone, and then to talk about him, or let the conversation develop in generalities? If this does occur and if he goes away, finishing the call without having mentioned the deceased, will there be some later reaction-pattern of guilt?

DR. LIEBMAN: I would say now that I used to do things the wrong way; I try now to do them the right way. Our usual approach has been to divert the bereaved person from his loss by talking about many extraneous events. Laymen will continue to pursue this method, but clergymen should, it seems to me, help the bereaved to verbalize their deep sense of loss. There is a kind of healing process that goes on when we as ministers allow the grief-stricken to talk to us about the virtues of the one who has departed. That very discussion is therapeutic.

Now I know that we are very uncomfortable in the presence of tears because we have all been affected by the stoicism of the Anglo-Saxon tradition. Yet the research work carried on by Dr. Lindemann and his associates indicates that this stoicism often can become the enemy of mental health. Not that people should force themselves to express grief when they genuinely do not feel it. When an old friend, for example, who has been painfully suffering from some incurable disease finds release through the Angel of Death, we do not usually experience prolonged grief or rebellion. Of course, even in such a situation where death has come as a blessed escape from terrible anguish, if we feel deep sorrow we should express it. We should always be free to pour forth our emotions in grief if we feel them. The worst thing to do is to deny your grief in conformity with certain conventions in Western culture.

Honesty is the best policy in the realm of sorrow as in every other realm. We must learn not to deny our real emotions of joy or of tragedy.

We ministers can be of tremendous help to our parishoners if we encourage them to express to us what is genuinely in their hearts and if in our visits with them after the death of a loved one we provide both the listening ear and the friendly interacting spirit with whom they can begin to take up the threads of life once again.

DR. BREWSTER: I certainly agree with Dr. Liebman. There is no satisfactory substitute for grief except grieving. Any method which helps the bereaved complete his grief work is legitimate. The only danger of our efforts as minister or psychiatrist is that they will fail to save the bereaved from becoming a victim of the symptoms and sequellae of morbid grief. The goal which grieving persons uniformly welcome is emancipation not from all traces of memory but from the crippling emotional bondage to the deceased.